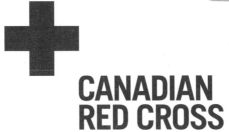

**CANADIAN
RED CROSS**

First Aid & CPR
Manual

This manual belongs to:

_____

StayWell

StayWell

This publication is available in English and French.

The terms he and she have been used throughout the manual to ensure representation of both genders and to correspond to any photos within a particular section.

Glossary terms are bolded in green.

Illustrations by Jackie Wald
Printing/binding in Canada by Transcontinental

The StayWell Health Company Ltd.
2 Quebec Street, Suite 107, Guelph ON N1H 2T3
A part of
Krames StayWell Strategic Partnerships Division
780 Township Line Road, Yardley, PA 19067-4200 USA

ISBN: 978-1-58480-513-7

16 17 18 19 / 10 9 8 7

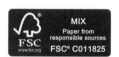

Contents

Acknowledgements

Over the past 65 years, the Canadian Red Cross First Aid Programs have developed and grown. Each time a program is revised, its foundation is built on the great work completed in the previous revision. We would like to acknowledge everyone who worked on the programs and products before us.

This project was completed because of the creative vision and dedication of the Canadian Red Cross National Medical Advisory Committee (NMAC) and the Canadian Red Cross National First Aid Technical Advisory Group.

NMAC reviewed the content of the program. The committee was made up of Andrew MacPherson (chair), MD, CCFP-EM, and Brendan J. Hughes, MD, CCFP.

The Canadian Red Cross National First Aid Technical Advisory Group was responsible for providing overall leadership, dedication, and direction. The group includes Bev Glass (chair), Patrick Boucher, Rob Briscoe, Blair Doyle, Dominique Graf, Kevin Holder, Jeff Horseman, Sioban Kennedy, Jason Oliver, Julie Poirier, Kathy Sampson, and Kevin Sanford.

The Canadian Association of Wound Care was pleased to review Chapter 8, Wound Care, of this manual.

The Canadian Athletic Therapists Association and the Canadian Council of Snowmobile Organizations were pleased to review Chapter 9, Head and Spine Injuries, of this manual.

The Canadian Medical Association and SMARTRISK are pleased to support the important work of the Canadian Red Cross in developing this *First Aid & CPR Manual*.

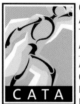

CANADIAN
ATHLETIC
THERAPISTS
ASSOCIATION

ASSOCIATION
CANADIENNE
DES THÉRAPEUTES
DU SPORT

CATA

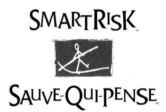

SMARTRISK

SAUVE-QUI-PENSE

Canadian Association
of Wound Care

Association canadienne
du soin des plaies

ASSOCIATION
MÉDICALE
CANADIENNE

CANADIAN
MEDICAL
ASSOCIATION

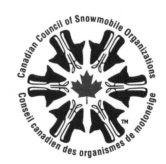

The Fundamental Principles of the International Red Cross and Red Crescent Movement

Humanity
The International Red Cross and Red Crescent Movement, born of a desire to bring assistance without discrimination to the wounded on the battlefield, endeavours, in its international and national capacity, to prevent and alleviate human suffering wherever it may be found. Its purpose is to protect life and health and ensure respect for the human being. It promotes mutual understanding, friendship, co-operation, and lasting peace amongst all peoples.

Impartiality
It makes no discrimination as to nationality, race, religious beliefs, class, or political opinions. It endeavours to relieve the suffering of individuals, being guided solely by their needs, and to give priority to the most urgent cases of distress.

Neutrality
In order to continue to enjoy the confidence of all, the Movement may not take sides in hostilities or engage at any time in controversies of a political, racial, religious, or ideological nature.

Independence
The Movement is independent. The National Societies, while auxiliaries in the humanitarian services of their governments and subject to the laws of their respective countries, must always maintain their autonomy so that they may be able at all times to act in accordance with the principles of the Movement.

Voluntary Service
It is a voluntary relief movement not prompted in any manner by desire for gain.

Unity
There can be only one Red Cross or one Red Crescent Society in any one country. It must be open to all. It must carry on its humanitarian work throughout its territory.

Universality
The International Red Cross and Red Crescent Movement, in which all Societies have equal status and share equal responsibilities and duties in helping each other, is worldwide.

The Fundamental Principles were proclaimed by the XXth International Conference of the Red Cross, Vienna, 1965. This is the revised text contained in the Statutes of the International Red Cross and the Red Crescent Movement, adopted by the XXVth International Conference of the Red Cross, Geneva, 1986.

In keeping with the Fundamental Principles of the Red Cross, the Society is committed to Social Justice in the elimination of Society structures and actions that oppress, exclude, limit, or discriminate on the basis of race, gender, ethnicity, financial ability, sexual orientation, religion, disability, or age.

The Canadian Red Cross Society

Founded 1896

Incorporated 1909

The red cross emblem and designation "Red Cross" are reserved in Canada by law for the exclusive use of The Canadian Red Cross Society and for the medical units of the armed forces by the Geneva Conventions Act, R.S.C., 1985, c. G-3.

The programs of The Canadian Red Cross Society are made possible by the voluntary services and financial support of the Canadian people.

LOCAL EMERGENCY NUMBERS

EMS: _____

Fire: _____

Ambulance: _____

Police: _____

Poison Control Centre: _____

LOCAL RED CROSS TELEPHONE NUMBER

_____

The Red Cross

The Red Cross

The year is 1859. You are a soldier in the French army, and you have been severely wounded. As blood spurts from a bullet hole in your thigh, you collapse onto the battlefield. You assume that you will die. Later, however, you find yourself confused but alive, lying next to an enemy soldier from the Austrian army. You are no longer on the battlefield, and strangers are tending to your wounds as well as those of your comrades and your enemies. You are too grateful to be alive to think about war any longer.

HENRY DUNANT—The Red Cross Founder

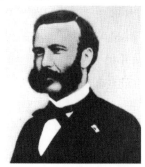

Figure 1.1 Henry Dunant.

- In June 1859, Henry Dunant (Figure 1.1) saw an unforgettable scene: 40,000 dead and wounded soldiers left on the field after the Battle of Solferino in Italy.

- Dunant organized local villagers into first aid teams to help as many of the wounded as possible, saving thousands of lives.

NOTE:

In December of 2005, the International Red Cross and Red Crescent Movement welcomed the decision to create an additional emblem alongside the red cross and red crescent, the red crystal.

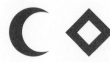

- To prevent this horror from happening again, he decided to create a neutral organization to care for wounded soldiers and prisoners—an organization that would be respected and protected by both sides in any conflict. The result was the Red Cross.

- Dunant spent the rest of his life trying to reduce the suffering caused by war. He lobbied governments, organized Red Cross Societies in different countries, and spoke to the public.

- Today, the symbol chosen for the Red Cross is recognized around the world: a red cross on a white background.

- In 1901, Dunant won the first Nobel Peace Prize. By founding the International Red Cross and Red Crescent Movement, he has saved the lives of millions of people over the years.

On May 19, 1909, Parliament passed the Canadian Red Cross Society Act, which established the Canadian Red Cross to serve Canadians as an auxiliary to government and the public authority, in accordance with the Geneva Conventions. (Prior to 1909, it operated as a branch of the British Red Cross.) As a result, for more than a century, Canadians have had their own national Red Cross Society dedicated to improving the situations of the most vulnerable people in Canada and around the world.

THE RED CROSS—The Fundamental Principles

There are Red Cross or Red Crescent Societies in more than 190 countries around the world.

In every country, our programs and activities are guided by seven Fundamental Principles. The Tanzanian Red Cross has created a short, simple version of these principles:

Humanity: We serve people, but not systems.

Impartiality: We care for the victims and the aggressors alike.

Neutrality: We take initiatives, but never take sides.

Independence: We bow to needs, but not rulers.

Voluntary Service: We work around the clock, but never for personal gain.

Unity: We have many talents, but a single idea.

Universality: We respect nations, but our work knows no bounds.

Essentially, we provide help to people in need, whatever their race, political beliefs, religion, social status, or culture.

WHO WE ARE—The Canadian Red Cross

 ### Our Mission

The Canadian Red Cross's mission is to improve the lives of vulnerable people by mobilizing the power of humanity in Canada and around the world.

 ### Our Vision

The Canadian Red Cross is the leading humanitarian organization through which people voluntarily demonstrate their caring for others in need.

 ### Our Values

Our actions and decisions are based on:

- humanitarian values;
- respect, dignity, and care for one another within and outside the Canadian Red Cross; and
- integrity, accountability, effectiveness, and transparency.

 ### Our Volunteers

Volunteers are the heart of the Canadian Red Cross. More than 25,000 Red Cross volunteers give their time and energy to help others every day. If you are looking for opportunities to give back to your community, meet new people, have new experiences, learn new skills, or to develop your professional skills training, volunteering for the Canadian Red Cross is the right choice for you.

HOW WE HELP

 ### Disaster Management

The Canadian Red Cross helps people affected by emergencies and disasters. We work with governments and with other humanitarian organizations to meet people's basic needs. We provide food, clothing, shelter, first aid, and emotional support. When families have been separated by disasters, we help bring them back together.

 ### International Operations

The Canadian Red Cross works in other countries to help people who have been affected by wars and natural disasters. We bring urgently needed supplies, reunite families, and help rebuild communities. Each year, we send about 100 professional relief workers on overseas missions.

 ### First Aid Programs

The Canadian Red Cross First Aid Programs have been training Canadians in first aid for the past 65 years. Our courses give people the knowledge and skills to deal with emergency situations and to prevent injuries from happening.

 ### Swimming and Water Safety Program

Since 1946, more than 32 million Canadians have learned how to swim and safely enjoy water activities with the Canadian Red Cross. Our Red Cross Swim programs are unique because they consider each swimmer's individual needs and offer participants of all abilities and ages (preschool, kids, teens, and adults) opportunities to learn swimming and water safety skills. Teens and adults can also enjoy aquatic sports and enrol in lifeguarding courses.

 ### RespectED: Violence and Abuse Prevention

Since 1984, in communities across the country, the Canadian Red Cross has been helping to break the cycle of hurt. RespectED: Violence and Abuse Prevention programs promote healthier relationships and safer communities through education and partnerships.

 ### Homecare Services

The Canadian Red Cross provides in-home community services to help individuals in Ontario and Atlantic Canada live as independently as possible. The services enhance people's well-being and dignity, be they frail or elderly, children at risk, people with disabilities, or palliative patients.

Health Equipment Loan Programs (HELP)

For more than 50 years, the Canadian Red Cross has been offering Health Equipment Loan Programs (HELP) that allow Canadians throughout much of the country to borrow basic health and mobility devices such as wheelchairs or walkers. More than 200,000 Canadians make use of this service each year, lessening the burden on families already coping with injury or illness.

NOTES:

Preparing to Respond

Preparing to Respond

You are the first to arrive at the scene of a motor vehicle collision. There are two people involved. A woman is sitting by the side of the road with a large cut on her leg, which is bleeding severely. A man is lying on the ground moaning and coughing.

First aid is the immediate care that you give to an ill or injured person until more advanced care can be obtained.

LEVELS OF FIRST AID TRAINING

There are different levels of first aid training:

Emergency first aid deals with life-threatening conditions. It focuses on airway, breathing, and circulation emergencies and wounds (chapters 1 to 8).

Standard first aid deals with life-threatening conditions and with emergencies that could lead to life-threatening situations if they are not treated (chapters 1 to 13). It focuses on:

- Airway, breathing, and circulation emergencies
- Wounds
- Head and spine injuries
- Injuries to bones, muscles, and joints
- Sudden medical emergencies
- Heat-related and cold-related emergencies
- Poisonings

THE FIRST AIDER'S ROLE

Your role includes three basic steps:

1. Recognize the emergency.
2. Call emergency medical services (EMS)/9-1-1.
3. Act according to your skills, knowledge, and comfort level.

RECOGNIZE AN EMERGENCY

The first step in dealing with an emergency is to recognize it:

- A **medical emergency** is an illness or condition that needs immediate medical attention. For example, a heart attack is a medical emergency.

- An **injury** is some kind of damage to the body caused by an external force. This damage can include broken **bones**, wounds, and burns. The most common causes of injuries include motor vehicle collisions, falls, poisonings, and drownings. Some injuries are serious enough to be considered emergencies. If you're not sure, call EMS/9-1-1 and let the professionals decide.

PREPARE! STAY SAFE! SURVIVE!

- **Prepare!** includes everything you do before you start an activity, including taking a first aid or **cardiopulmonary resuscitation (CPR)** course. Carry first aid kits and supplies.

- **Stay Safe!** includes everything you do during the activity, such as wearing the proper safety gear. Follow safe work practices and procedures.

- **Survive!** includes actions you take to ensure the safety and the survival of yourself and others, such as identifying and reporting hazards in your workplace, home, and community or providing first aid in an emergency.

> **REMEMBER:**
>
> Injuries are not accidents. Injuries are predictable and preventable.
>
> Planning for safety is the best way to prevent injuries.
>
> Good First Aiders keep safe and make wise choices. They help teach friends and family about making wise choices as well.

DECIDE TO ACT

Many lives are saved because people like you get involved. Every year many **bystanders** in Canada recognize and respond to emergencies. Some phone for help, some comfort the ill or injured person or family members, some give first aid, and some help keep order at the emergency scene.

One of the simplest and most important ways of providing first aid is to call for help (EMS/9-1-1). By making this call, you'll make sure that highly trained medical professionals arrive to care for the ill or injured person (Figure 2.1).

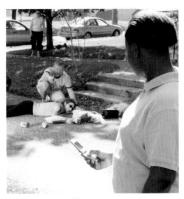

Figure 2.1 Call EMS/9-1-1.

BARRIERS TO ACTION

Sometimes people don't want to get involved in an emergency for various reasons. The five most common concerns are:

1. **Other people at the scene:** If there are other people at the scene, it's easy to think that they can take care of the emergency without your help. However, you should never assume that someone is providing first aid just because you see a lot of people. And remember that there are many important jobs that you can do. You can help control the crowd, call EMS/9-1-1, get supplies, or comfort the ill or injured person.

2. **The ill or injured person:** You may not feel comfortable treating people if they are behaving oddly, if they are much older or younger than you, or if they are of a different race or gender. Remember, whoever they are, they need help.

3. **Unpleasant injuries or illnesses:** You may feel upset or sick when you see blood, vomit, broken bones, or other injuries. If this happens, take a few deep breaths to help calm yourself before you deal with the situation.

4. **Catching a disease:** You might have a concern that you could catch something from the injured person. There are many ways to reduce the risks, and we'll discuss them in this chapter. If you take simple precautions while performing first aid, you can limit the possibility of catching a serious disease.

5. **Doing something wrong:** You might be afraid of getting sued if you make a mistake. As long as you act reasonably and carefully, you don't need to worry. All provinces and territories have laws to protect bystanders who give emergency help. Use your good judgment and don't try to do something that you're not trained to do. Once you start giving first aid, keep providing help until emergency medical services (EMS) personnel arrive.

Thinking about these things now and mentally preparing yourself for an emergency will help you overcome your fears.

GET CONSENT

Once you decide to act, get the ill or injured person's consent. To get **consent**, tell the person three things:

1. Who you are
2. That you are trained in first aid
3. That you are here to help

If a **baby** or a **child** is ill or injured:

- Ask the supervising adult for consent.
- If the baby or child is alone, you can assume you have consent to give first aid.

NOTE:

If the person is unconscious, consent is implied.

If the person refuses your help:

- Have someone call EMS/9-1-1. Let them know the person has refused help. The EMS personnel who arrive will deal with the situation.
- Do not try to give the person help by force.
- Stay nearby if possible.

PREPARING FOR EMERGENCIES

By being prepared for emergencies, you can make sure that an ill or injured person gets help as soon as possible. First aid training gives you a plan of action for any emergency and gives you the confidence to act.

After you have learned first aid, stay prepared for emergencies by practising regularly and keeping your certifications up to date. Think of emergencies that could happen in your home or workplace and rehearse how you would respond. Make sure your family and co-workers know what to do in all types of emergencies. Suggest that they take a first aid course too.

PREPARING FOR EMERGENCIES AT HOME

- Keep important information about you and your family in a handy place. Include your address, everyone's date of birth, health card numbers, medical conditions, allergies, and prescriptions and dosages. List the names and phone numbers of your doctors.

- Keep your medical records up to date.

- Post the numbers for the police, fire department, EMS, and **Poison Control Centre** near every phone in your home.

- Teach children how to call for help.

- Install smoke and carbon monoxide detectors. Test them regularly.

- Keep an up-to-date first aid kit handy in your home, car, and workplace.

- Learn and practise first aid skills such as CPR.

- Make sure your house or apartment number is easy to see.

- You should wear a **MedicAlert® medical identification product** if you have a potentially serious medical condition such as **seizures**, diabetes, heart disease, or allergies.

AFTER AN EMERGENCY

After dealing with an emergency it is often helpful to talk to somebody about the situation. If you are really affected, you can contact your local crisis intervention line or look in your phone book for information on whom to contact.

As a **First Aider** you can help others involved in the emergency by talking to them and providing comfort.

PREPARING FOR DISASTERS

Disasters and personal emergencies can, and do, happen anywhere in Canada.

The key to being prepared is to identify what disasters could happen in your home, workplace, and recreational area.

To prepare for emergencies and disasters in the workplace, follow your employer's protocol.

PREPARING FOR DISASTERS AT HOME

- Talk with your family about the dangers of fire, severe weather, and other emergencies that could happen in your area.
- Pick two meeting places—one near your home to use in case of fire and one outside the neighbourhood to use in case you cannot return home after a disaster.
- Keep family records in a waterproof and fireproof container.
- Have emergency supply kits handy.
- Call the Canadian Red Cross for disaster education program information or visit our website at www.redcross.ca.

AFTER A DISASTER

- Move people away from unsafe areas.
- Unless you need to call EMS/9-1-1, don't use the telephone.
- If you have been separated from your family, register with the local Red Cross.
- If you have to evacuate your home, wear sturdy shoes and clothing that will keep you comfortable. Take your emergency supplies kit. Lock your home when you leave and use the travel routes that local officials recommend.

INFECTION

An **infection** is a disease process caused by germs that invade your body. For someone to get an infection or infectious disease, four things must happen:

1. Germs must be present in the surrounding environment.
2. The germs must enter the body.
3. Enough germs must be present in the body to cause infection.
4. The individual's natural defences must be weak.

If any one of these is missing, you won't get an infection. For example, germs present on your **skin** cannot harm you if they cannot enter your body. If you are immune to a particular disease because you have received a vaccination, your immune system will kill the germs in your body that cause the particular disease before you become infected.

Knowing how germs are spread will help you understand how to prevent infection.

How Is an Infection Spread From One Person to Another?

There are four different ways that infections can be spread from one person to another (disease transmission):

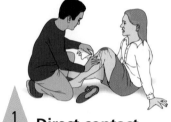

1 Direct contact

—for example, when you touch the blood of someone who is infected.

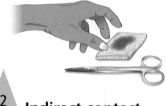

2 Indirect contact

—for example, when you pick up something that an infected person has touched.

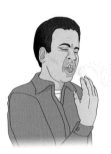

3 Airborne transmission

—for example, when an infected person sneezes, sending germs into the air, and you breathe in those germs.

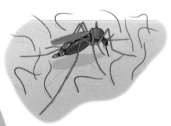

4 Vector-borne transmission

—for example, when a mosquito bites an infected person and then bites you, passing on the germs.

Some infections are spread through only one of these routes. Others may be spread through several routes.

How to Prevent Diseases From Spreading

There are some basic precautions that you can take to stop diseases from spreading:

Type of Precaution	Definition	Example
Personal Precautions	Actions that individuals can take to reduce the risk of spreading disease	Wash your hands frequently and thoroughly. See "Handwashing" in this chapter. Treat all blood and other body fluids as infectious materials. Cover your mouth and nose when you sneeze. Eat well and get enough exercise and sleep.
Equipment Precautions	Items that protect you from direct contact with contaminated objects	Always use some type of barrier device between you and any material that could be infected. Wear safety glasses, goggles, masks, gloves (choose non-latex or safety gloves), and any other personal protective equipment your workplace specifies. If there is a chance you might get splashed with body fluids, wear safety glasses or a face shield. Use **dressings** to minimize your contact with blood. **NOTE:** You must use personal protective equipment in the workplace. However, if you are helping a family member, it is your choice whether you use personal protective equipment.
Environmental Precautions	The set-up of an area that reduces exposure to germs	Make sure there is proper ventilation in your workplace. Make sure that people don't use the same sink for hygiene and food preparation. Dispose of any contaminated materials immediately. **NOTE:** Many environmental precautions are the responsibility of the employer, but you can make suggestions if you notice something could be improved.

▶ Handwashing

Handwashing is an important precaution wherever you are. It helps prevent you from spreading germs that can cause many infectious diseases. Use the following guidelines for washing your hands:

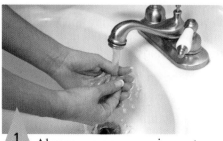

1 Always use warm running water and a mild soap.

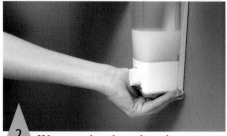

2 Wet your hands and apply some soap (use liquid soap if possible; antibacterial soap is optional).

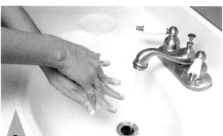

3 Rub your hands together vigorously until you see a soapy lather. Keep rubbing your hands for at least 20 to 30 seconds. Make sure you scrub between your fingers, under your fingernails, and around the backs and palms of your hands.

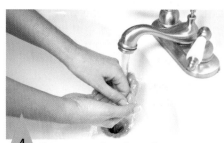

4 Rinse your hands under warm running water. Leave the water running while you dry your hands.

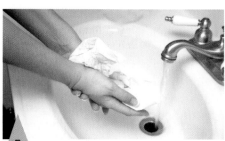

5 Dry your hands with a clean, disposable towel. Be careful not to touch the faucet handles or the towel holder with your clean hands.

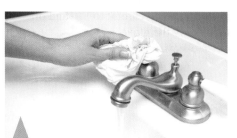

6 Turn the faucet off using the towel as a barrier between your hands and the faucet handle. Use it as a barrier for the door handle as well. Throw the towel into a trash can.

You should wash your hands:

- Before and after contact with an ill or injured person
- After removing gloves
- After helping in an emergency
- When your hands look dirty
- Before eating or drinking
- After handling dirty articles, instruments, or dressings
- Before or after treating wounds
- Before going home from work

Hand sanitizers and alcohol hand-rubs are appropriate for rapidly decontaminating your hands if they are otherwise clean. They are not a substitute for handwashing if your hands are soiled. When you can see dirt on your hands, you should first wash them with soap and water.

▶ Gloves

When you take off a pair of gloves, make sure that the outside of the glove doesn't touch your skin. Always wash your hands after you take off gloves.

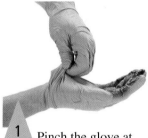
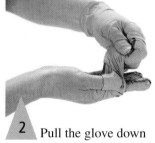
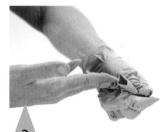

1 Pinch the glove at the wrist, being careful to touch only the glove's outside surface.

2 Pull the glove down and off.

3 Form the glove into a ball and hold it in the other hand. Insert thumb under inside rim of other glove, on palm side, then push glove inside out and down onto fingers and over balled glove. Discard gloves appropriately.

Some people are allergic to latex. For some people, latex causes a mild skin rash. For others, it can cause a life-threatening reaction called **anaphylaxis**. When you're giving first aid, always check for MedicAlert® medical identification products that will tell you if the person has a serious illness or allergy.

Immunization

Most people have been immunized against common childhood diseases such as measles and mumps (Figure 2.2). **Immunization** introduces a substance into your body that builds up your resistance against the germs that cause a specific disease.

Children usually get immunizations because these are required for school or sports programs. However, not all adults have been immunized. Talk to your doctor or local community health nurse about your immunizations.

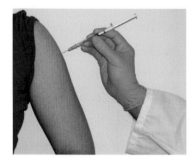

Figure 2.2 Immunization helps prevent illness and disease.

If you are planning a trip outside the country, find out long before you plan to travel which immunizations you need for the countries you will visit.

Immunizations not only protect you, they also protect your family, friends, and co-workers.

Because the risk of disease varies from place to place, this manual cannot cover all the hazards that you might face. For specific guidelines on your particular situation, talk to your doctor or call your community public health centre.

The Emergency Medical Services System

The Emergency Medical Services System

While you're driving on a rural road, the car in front of you suddenly goes off the road and rolls into a ditch. You see that the airbag has deployed, so you pull over and then reach for your cellphone.

The **emergency medical services (EMS) system** is a network of community resources and personnel organized to give emergency care in cases of injury or sudden illness. It varies from community to community. In many areas you can call 9-1-1, whereas other areas have a different local number. The level of training of the EMS personnel may also vary.

WHO IS COMING TO HELP?

There are several different kinds of trained personnel who may respond after you call for help.

First Responders: These include police, firefighters, or job-specific personnel such as athletic trainers or industrial safety personnel (Figure 3.1).

Paramedics: These are highly specialized emergency personnel who can often administer medications, including medications that are given intravenously (through IVs) in some cases. They provide the highest level of pre-hospital care.

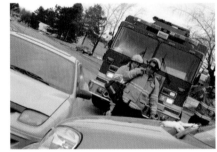

Figure 3.1 A first responder in action.

WHEN TO CALL EMS/9-1-1

Trust your instincts. If you think that an emergency exists, it probably does. Do not lose time calling friends or family members—call EMS/9-1-1 for professional help immediately. It is better for these professionals to come and find out they are not needed than not to come in an emergency when they were needed.

You should call EMS/9-1-1 in cases of:

- Danger to you or to others
- Unconsciousness or an altered level of consciousness
- Difficulty breathing or no signs of breathing
- Persistent chest pain or pressure
- Deadly bleeding
- Seizures, severe headache, or slurred speech
- Injuries to the head and/or spine
- Blood in the vomit, urine, or stool
- Imminent childbirth

In addition to the cases listed above, you should call EMS/9-1-1 if the ill or injured person is involved in, or exposed to, the following:

- Fire or explosion
- Poisonous gas
- Swift-moving water

- Motor vehicle collision
- Live electrical wires
- A situation where you cannot get to the ill or injured person easily

Contact your local Poison Control Centre for any suspected poisoning.

HOW TO CALL EMS/9-1-1

When you call, the EMS dispatcher who answers will likely ask:

- Where is the emergency?
- What telephone number are you calling from?
- What is your name?
- What has happened?
- How many people are involved and what is their condition?

Don't hang up until the dispatcher tells you to.

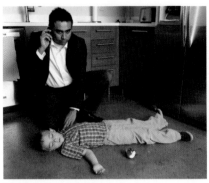

Figure 3.2 Call EMS/9-1-1 when you are alone.

Sending someone else to call the emergency number is better than calling it yourself because it means that you can stay with the ill or injured person and keep giving first aid. If you are alone with the person, call out loudly for help. If no one comes, get to a phone as quickly as you can to call EMS/9-1-1 (Figure 3.2). As soon as you hang up, return to the person to keep giving help.

If someone else can make the call for you, ask that person to come back and tell you what the EMS/9-1-1 dispatcher said. If that person has a cellphone, he or she can stay with you.

Cellphones and other electronic devices can display emergency contacts. The letters "ICE" (In Case of Emergency) may appear in the phone's contacts list next to the name of a doctor, spouse, or other important contact. If the person has programmed his or her ICE contact with a "0" in front, it will appear as the first contact in the list.

 Should You Drive an Ill or Injured Person to Hospital?

Never try to drive an ill or injured person anywhere yourself if the condition is life-threatening or if it might become life-threatening, such as chest pain, which may lead to cardiac arrest. Instead, call EMS/9-1-1 and wait for help. A car or boat trip may make things worse for the person.

If the person is a friend or family member, and if you are sure the person's injuries are minor, you may decide to take the person to a hospital, doctor's office, or nursing station yourself. It can be a good idea to call the hospital or doctor's office and let them know you are on your way with an ill or injured person. Take someone else with you to help keep the person comfortable and to watch for any changes in the person's condition.

Never let an ill or injured person drive alone to get help. If the person's condition gets worse, it could be unsafe to drive.

MOVING A PERSON BEFORE PROVIDING CARE

Move an ill or injured person only if:

- The person's position stops you from giving care for a life-threatening injury or illness.

- The ill or injured person is blocking access to someone with a more serious injury or illness.

- The person is likely to drown.

- The scene is becoming unsafe.

▶ Clothes Drag

To move someone who may have a head and/or spine injury:

1. Hold the person's clothing behind the person's neck.

2. Pull the person to safety.

3. While moving the person, cradle the head with the person's clothes and your hands. Keep the person's head, neck, and back in a straight line as best as you can.

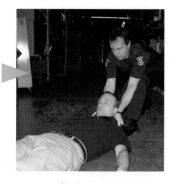

▶ Two-Person Seat Carry

To carry someone who cannot walk and isn't likely to have a head and/or spine injury:

1. Stand on one side of the person and have another First Aider stand on the other side.

2. Put one arm under the person's thighs and the other across the person's back while the other First Aider does the same thing.

3. Hold the other First Aider's wrists underneath the person's legs and across the person's back. Have the other First Aider hold your wrists.

4. Move the person to safety.

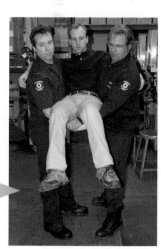

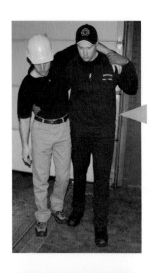

 ## Walking Assist

To move someone who needs help walking to safety:

1. Have the person stand up.

2. Stand on the person's weak or injured side and put his arm across your shoulders. Hold it there with one hand.

3. Support the person with your other hand around the waist.

4. Move the person to safety.

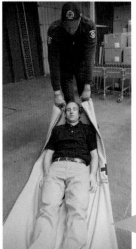

 ## Blanket Drag

To move someone in an emergency situation when you don't have a stretcher:

1. Keep the person between you and the blanket.

2. Gather half the blanket and place it against the person's side.

3. Roll the person towards you. Make sure the person's body moves as a unit.

4. Reach over and pull the blanket towards the person so that you can roll the person on top of it.

5. Roll the person back, onto the blanket.

6. Gather the blanket at the head and move the person to safety.

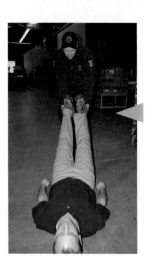

 ## Foot Drag

To move someone who cannot otherwise be carried or moved:

1. Firmly grasp the person's ankles and move backwards.

2. Pull the person in a straight line, being careful not to bump the person's head.

▶ Assisting a Conscious, Drowning Person With a Reaching Assist

To rescue someone who is far out in the water:

Have someone call EMS/9-1-1 and get an **automated external defibrillator (AED)**. If you are alone, call EMS/9-1-1 yourself, then get an AED. Call for a lifeguard or other trained person. You need special training to swim out to rescue someone. If you do not have proper training, entering the water to help a person is dangerous. The person may try to hold onto you and is likely to pull you under the water.

To rescue someone who is nearby in the water:

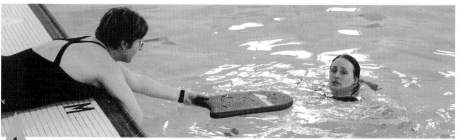

1 Find something that you can hold out to reach the person, such as a pole, oar or paddle, tree branch, shirt, belt, or towel.

Lie down in a safe position. The best position is lying down at a 45-degree angle to the side of the dock or pool with your legs spread out to keep you stable. Firmly brace yourself so that you won't get pulled into the water. If you can't lie down, crouch or bend on one knee, staying as far from the water's edge as you can.

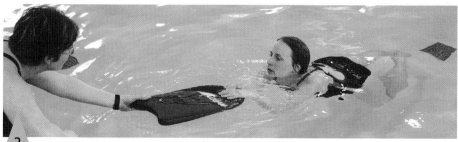

2 Hold out your reaching assist for the person to grab.

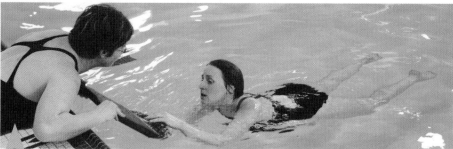

3 Pull the reaching assist back in and then move to the edge of the water to secure the person.

NOTES:

Check, Call, Care

Check, Call, Care

At the local playground, a three-year-old boy has fallen from the top of a slide and is lying on the ground, screaming in pain. You are one of three people trained in first aid to come to the scene and offer help.

The **primary survey** is an examination of the emergency scene and the ill or injured person for life-threatening conditions. It consists of three basics steps to follow in any emergency: **Check, Call, Care**.

PRIMARY SURVEY

 Check

Once you recognize an emergency, take time to look around and do the following before you begin to help:

Check the Scene

- Is it safe (Figure 4.1)? *Look* for things such as glass, hostile bystanders, or oncoming cars; *listen* for things such as alarms or escaping gas; and *smell* for things such as gas or smoke.

- What happened? How did it happen?

- How many ill or injured people are there?

- Is there someone to help me?

- Is there someone who looks to be **unconscious**?

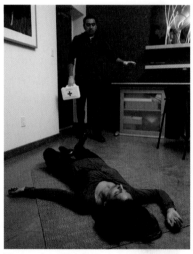

Figure 4.1 Check the scene for safety.

▶ When More Than One Person Is Ill or Injured

If you are ever in a situation where there are several ill or injured people, the general principle is to do what is best for the most people. This is called **triage**.

As an example, if someone has minor bleeding and another person has deadly bleeding, you should help the person with deadly bleeding because EMS personnel will arrive before the minor bleeding becomes serious. Deadly bleeding is life-threatening *right now*. If you have to decide who needs your help most urgently, trust your own judgment to do what is best for the most people.

Check the Person

1. If it is safe to do so, check the person (Figure 4.2):

   - Ask the person, "Are you okay?" Use the person's name if you know it.

   - If the person does not respond to your voice, tap the person on the shoulder.

2. Does the person want your help? Tell the person:

   - Who you are

   - That you are trained in first aid

   - That you are here to help

   If someone is unconscious or can't answer because of the illness or injury, you can assume you have consent to give first aid.

   Never risk your own safety. Leave dangerous situations for EMS personnel.

3. Check the person's **ABCs**: Airway, Breathing, and Circulation.

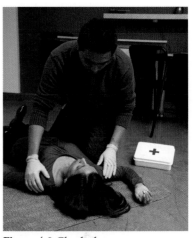

Figure 4.2 Check the person.

NOTE:

Instead of tapping a baby on the shoulder, clap loudly, and gently flick the bottom of the baby's feet.

A = CHECK THE AIRWAY / B = CHECK BREATHING

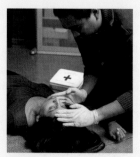

Figure 4.3 Open the airway.

> **NOTE:**
>
> Checking the ABCs is a rapid assessment that is done simultaneously and should take no more than 5 to 10 seconds.

Your first job is to make sure the person has an open **airway**. The airway is the pathway from the mouth and nose to the **lungs**. If it is closed or obstructed, air cannot get in, making it impossible to breathe. Anyone who can speak or cry has an open airway.

If the person is unconscious, you must make sure the airway is open. To do this, tilt the head back and lift the chin (Figure 4.3). This action, called the **head-tilt/chin-lift**, moves the tongue away from the back of the throat and lets air reach the lungs.

You'll learn more about dealing with airway emergencies in Chapter 5.

Next, check for breathing. Someone who can speak or cry is breathing.

Check for **normal breathing** for a maximum of 5 to 10 seconds (Figure 4.4). *Look* at an unconscious person carefully for signs of normal breathing. The chest should rise and fall. If there is only an occasional gasp of air (agonal respiration), the person is not breathing normally.

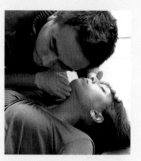

Figure 4.4 Check for normal breathing.

> **NOTE:**
>
> To assess normal breathing, put your face close to the person's face so that you can hear and feel air coming out of the person's nose and mouth while you watch the chest rising and falling.

C = CHECK CIRCULATION

Checking circulation (Figure 4.5) means looking for deadly bleeding and signs of shock (e.g., paler than normal skin colour, cool moist skin). Quickly look at the person from head to toe. Deadly bleeding must be controlled as soon as possible. You will learn how to do this in Chapter 6.

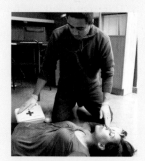

Figure 4.5 Check circulation.

If the person is breathing normally (more than an occasional gasp), it means that the **heart** is beating. However, if the person is not breathing normally, the heart may soon stop, so you should start **compressions**. You will learn how to do this in Chapter 7.

Call

An ill or injured person may have an altered level of consciousness. The person may be unresponsive to your voice or confused about time and place.

- If the person responds, determine whether there is any need to call EMS/9-1-1.

- If the person is unresponsive, have someone call EMS/9-1-1 and get an AED if available (Figure 4.6).

- If you are alone:

  ▶ For an adult, call EMS/9-1-1 yourself, get an AED, and return to care for the person (e.g., start CPR).

  ▶ For a child, do five cycles (two minutes) of CPR first, if necessary, then call EMS/9-1-1, get an AED, and return to care for the child.

  ▶ For a baby, do five cycles (two minutes) of CPR first, if necessary. Then take the baby with you (as long as you don't suspect a head and/or spine injury) to call EMS/9-1-1, get an AED, and return to providing care.

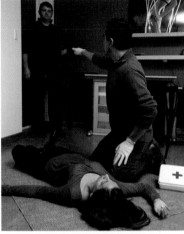

Figure 4.6 Have someone call EMS/9-1-1 and get an AED.

Care

Care for all life-threatening conditions first. (Treatment for life-threatening conditions is explained in the following chapters.)

NOTE:

Treat the person for shock if the ABCs are present.

NOTE:

If someone is there to help, he or she can treat deadly bleeding or treat for shock while you treat other life-threatening conditions.

H.A.IN.E.S. Recovery Position

Once you've checked the ABCs you should move an unconscious person into the **H.A.IN.E.S. recovery position** if:

1. You have to leave the person alone for any reason.

2. The person's airway is open.

3. The person is breathing.

4. There is no deadly bleeding.

The recovery position helps to keep the airway open and allows any blood or vomit to drain from the mouth, which is why it's also called the drainage position.

NOTE:	NOTE:	NOTE:
Ensure the injured person's head remains in contact with her outstretched arm and is supported by your hand.	H.A.IN.E.S. stands for High Arm In Endangered Spine.	If you need to leave the person alone to call EMS/9-1-1 and get an AED, roll the person into the H.A.IN.E.S. recovery position first.

To move someone into the recovery position if the person is on her back:

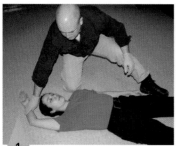

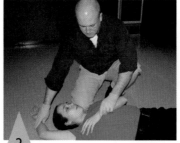

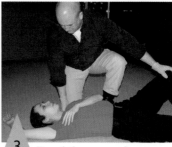

1 Kneel beside the person's waist. Raise the person's farthest arm away from you by rotating it outwards, while keeping the palm facing upwards.

2 Place the arm nearest to you across the person's chest, with fingers pointing to the opposite shoulder.

3 Bend the person's nearest leg at the knee.

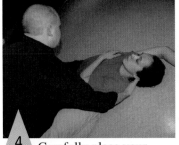

4 Carefully place your forearm—the one that is nearest to the person's head and neck—under the person's shoulder to provide extra leverage. Place the hand of that arm under the hollow of the person's neck and head to stabilize the person. DO NOT push or lift the person's head or neck.

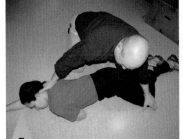

5 Carefully roll the person away from you by pushing simultaneously on the person's nearest shoulder with your stabilizing forearm and on the person's flexed knee with your other hand.

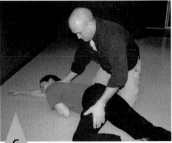

6 Pull the person's top leg closer to the chest.

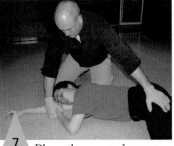

7 Place the person's upper hand on the outstretched arm against the forehead.

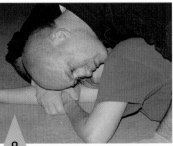

8 Check the person's airway and, if required, clear the airway with the face turned slightly downwards to permit drainage from the mouth.

9 Treat the person for shock, ensure the ABCs are present, and monitor the quality of the person's vital signs.

SHOCK

Shock happens when the vital organs do not get enough oxygen-rich blood. It is a very common condition that can affect the people involved in an emergency situation. Treat shock very seriously: it can be fatal.

Bystanders and First Aiders can be affected by emotional shock. Although this condition is not fatal, you should watch for it and treat it if it occurs.

 ## Common Causes

You should be on the lookout for shock with any injury, sudden illness, or involvement in a serious incident.

It is often caused by:

- Too much blood loss
- Extensive burns
- Too much fluid loss—because of diarrhea and vomiting for example, especially in children
- A weak heart
- Infection
- Emotion due to the impact of an event

 ## What to Look For

- Anxiety
- Skin that is paler than normal
- Confusion
- Rapid breathing
- Nausea and vomiting
- Cool, clammy skin
- Weakness
- Excessive thirst
- Drowsiness or loss of consciousness

What to Do

While you are waiting for EMS personnel to arrive:

1 Care for the cause of the shock.

2 Have the person rest.

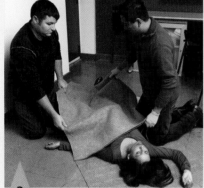

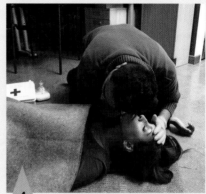

3 Keep the person warm.

4 Ensure the person's ABCs are present.

5 Give comfort and reassurance to the person.

SECONDARY SURVEY

If the person's ABCs are present, you need to find out what else may be wrong. To do this, you should do a **secondary survey** of the person to look for injuries that are not life-threatening at this point in time. There are three parts to this:

1. Ask questions. Interview the person (if he or she is **conscious**) and other people at the scene to get more information.

2. Check the quality of **vital signs**. Check for consciousness, breathing, and skin colour and temperature.

Skin that is paler than usual and lips that are bluish indicate problems with circulation.

3. Check the person for injuries from head to toe.

NOTE:

Only move to a secondary survey if the person's ABCs are present.

If you can, write down what you find during the secondary survey or have someone else write it down or help you remember. When EMS personnel arrive, give them the notes or tell them what you learned.

Signs are signals of illness or injury that a First Aider can see, hear, or feel when checking the ill or injured person.

Symptoms are things the ill or injured person says that he or she feels.

 ### Ask Questions

Get more information by asking the SAMPLE questions:

S = Signs and symptoms

> Are there any cuts or bruises? How do you feel? Do you feel any pain? Does anything feel different?

A = Allergies

> Are you allergic to anything?

M = Medications

> Do you take any medicine? What is it for?

P = Past medical history

> Do you have any medical conditions such as heart disease or another illness? Has this happened before?

L = Last meal

> When did you last eat? What did you eat?

E = Events leading up to the emergency

> What happened?

Check the Quality of Vital Signs

Level of consciousness Is the person awake or sleepy? Does the person seem confused? Is the person responsive?

Breathing Listen for sounds. Is the breathing fast or slow, shallow or deep? Is breathing painful for the person?

Skin Is it dry or wet? Is it an unusual colour or temperature?

Head-to-Toe Check

The goal of a **head-to-toe check** is to look carefully and systematically for injuries that aren't life-threatening.

Remember:

- Be careful not to cause further injury!
- Start by telling the person what you are going to do and ask the person to stay still.
- Avoid touching any painful areas or having the person move any area that hurts.
- Watch the person's expressions.
- Look for a MedicAlert® medical identification product. This may tell you what might be wrong, whom to call for help, and what care to give.

A MedicAlert® medical identification product indicates that the person wearing it has a particular medical condition. In the event of an emergency or non-critical medical situation, MedicAlert® lets emergency responders and healthcare providers immediately access a member's medical record, 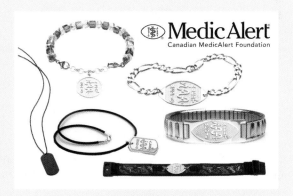 anytime and from anywhere in the world. These products include bracelets, necklaces, watch straps, wallet cards, and anklets. They can be silver or gold or in the form of a tattoo.

 Hands-Off Check

If the person is conscious and able to answer questions, do a **hands-off check**.

As you do this check, keep watching the person's level of consciousness, breathing, and skin colour. If any problems develop, stop whatever you are doing and give first aid *immediately*.

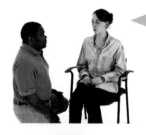

1 Start by telling the person what you are going to do and ask the person to stay still.

2 Look at all areas of the body that are not covered by clothing for discoloration (bruises) or deformities (odd shapes).

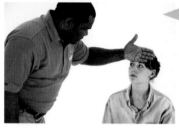

3 Look at the appearance of the skin and check its temperature with the back of your hand. A person with a breathing problem may have a face that is flushed or paler than normal. Cool, moist skin that is paler than normal often indicates shock. For privacy reasons, don't remove any articles of clothing from the person unless the clothing makes providing first aid difficult.

4 Ask the person to move each body part one at a time, beginning with the head, to see if anything hurts.

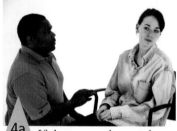

4a If the person has neck pain, do not move the neck. If there is no neck pain, ask if the person can slowly move her head from side to side.

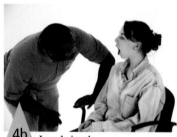

4b Look in the ears, nose, and mouth for blood or other fluids.

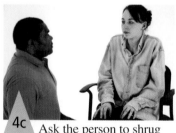

4c Ask the person to shrug her shoulders. Ask if there is any pain or discomfort.

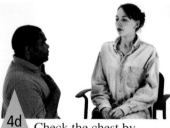

4d Check the chest by asking the person to take a deep breath and then blow the air out.

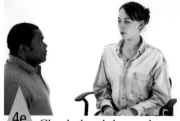

4e Check the abdomen by asking her to push her stomach out and then pull it in.

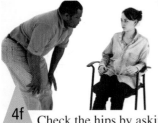

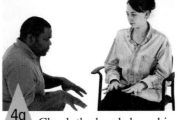

4f Check the hips by asking the person to move the hips slightly.

- If there is no pain in the hips, ask the person to wiggle the toes.
- If there is no pain in the toes, ask the person to move the ankles.
- If there is no pain in the ankles, ask the person to bend the knees.

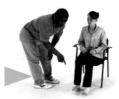

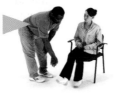

4g Check the hands by asking the person to wiggle the fingers.

- If there is no pain in the fingers, ask the person to move the wrists.
- If there is no pain in the wrists, ask the person to move the elbows.

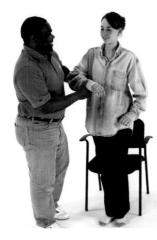

5 If the person doesn't complain of any pain and doesn't have any tender areas or signs of injury, ask the person to rest for a few minutes in a comfortable position. Check the quality of vital signs and ensure the person's ABCs are present. If you see no problem, help the person to stand up slowly when she is ready.

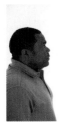

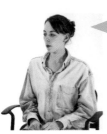

6 If the person has pain or dizziness or cannot move a body part, check the ABCs again. Have the person rest, help keep the body temperature normal, and give reassurance. If you find any injuries, provide first aid as needed and decide whether you need to call EMS/9-1-1.

Hands-On Check

You may need to do a **hands-on check** to assess whether further first aid is required. Do not perform a hands-on check unless you can be sure that the airway will not be compromised.

This check is mainly for an unconscious person who cannot tell you what is wrong. A conscious person will probably not like being touched. If the person is conscious, you may need to do a hands-on check at the site of the injury, but the entire check is not always necessary.

As you do this examination, keep watching the person's level of consciousness, breathing, and skin (vital signs). If any problems develop, *stop* whatever you are doing and give first aid *immediately*.

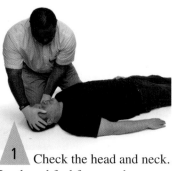

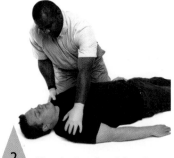

1 Check the head and neck. Look and feel for any abnormalities such as bumps, soft spots, or bleeding. Do not push on soft spots—they may be fractures of the skull.

2 Check the shoulders by looking and feeling for any bumps or bone deformities.

NOTE:	**NOTE:**	**NOTE:**
Remember to wear gloves when performing the hands-on check.	Do not continue to push or pull a body part if the person shows any signs of discomfort.	Be careful not to reach underneath someone because there could be glass or other objects that could hurt you. Look around and under the body for any signs of blood or fluids.

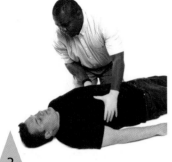

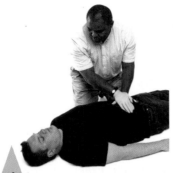

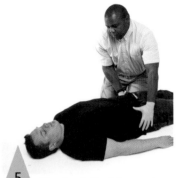

3 Check the chest by feeling the ribs for deformity. Ask the person to take a deep breath; both sides of the rib cage should expand at the same time. If any part of the ribs moves differently from the rest when the person breathes in or out, call EMS/9-1-1.

4 Gently press on the abdomen to see if it is hard.

- The abdomen should feel soft to the touch. If the abdomen is painful or hard to the touch, you may have to move or remove some of the person's clothing and check for bruising.

- Do not poke or push on a hard, painful, or bruised abdomen.

5 To check the hips, put your hands on both sides of the pelvis and push in and down on the hips at the same time. The hip bones should move together. Do not push or pull if the person shows any signs of discomfort.

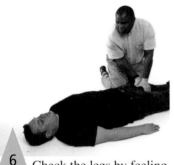

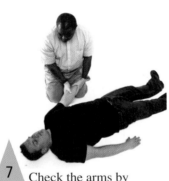

8 Complete all the steps of your secondary survey and then treat any injuries you have found. Treatment for various injuries is explained in the following chapters.

6 Check the legs by feeling for any deformity in the bones or any swelling.

7 Check the arms by feeling for any deformity in the bones or any swelling.

CONTINUAL CARE

After your secondary survey it is important to keep the person comfortable and ensure the ABCs are present until EMS personnel arrive.

Airway Emergencies

Airway Emergencies

At a family barbeque, your three-year-old nephew is finishing a hot dog as he runs over to join his older cousins, who are playing on a swing set. He starts to cough, so you go over to help. When you get close, he stops coughing, grabs his throat, and starts to turn blue.

The airway is the passage that connects the nose and mouth with the lungs. If anything blocks the airway (Figure 5.1), the person chokes and cannot get enough oxygen. This is a life-threatening condition, and you must give first aid to remove whatever is blocking the airway.

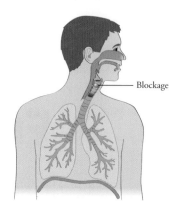

Blockage

Figure 5.1 A blockage in the airway.

MILD CHOKING

Coughing may indicate a mild **airway obstruction**. Coughing is a natural way to clear the airway, and it is a sign that the person is still getting enough air. Encourage the person to keep coughing and stay close by in case you need to help. An object may become more firmly stuck in the airway, stopping the person from breathing.

SEVERE CHOKING

Severe **choking** happens when a foreign object or swelling blocks the airway completely. The object may be stuck at any point in the airway from the throat to the lungs. This is a severe airway obstruction.

Common Causes

- Trying to swallow large pieces of food

- Eating while talking, walking, running, or playing

- Drinking too much alcohol before and during meals because alcohol affects **muscle** reflexes

Prevention

In adults:

- Chew food well before swallowing.

- Eat slowly and calmly.

- Do not talk, laugh, walk, or do other kinds of physical activity with food in your mouth.

- Do not drink too much alcohol before and during meals.

In children:

- Do not let young children walk, run, or play with food in their hands or mouth. Constantly watch children when they are eating.

- Feed babies or young children appropriate soft foods in small pieces.

- Make sure there are no small objects nearby that babies or young children could put in their mouth.

- Keep young children away from balloons, which can burst into small pieces that can be easily **inhaled**.

What to Look For

- Inability to speak, cough, or breathe

- Change in face colour (e.g., bluish or paler than normal)

- Look of panic with wide eyes

- One or both hands clutching the throat (Figure 5.2)

- High-pitched noises

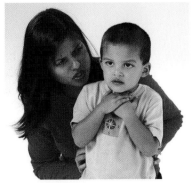

Figure 5.2 The universal sign for choking.

CONSCIOUS, CHOKING ADULT OR CHILD

 What to Do

Check:

- Check the scene to ensure it is safe.
- If it is safe to do so, check the person and the person's ABCs.

Call:

- Shout for help.

Care:

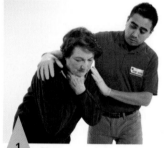

1 Encourage the person to continue coughing and do not interfere. The obstruction might clear itself.

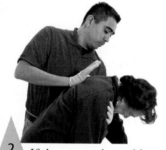

2 If the person is unable to speak, cough, or breathe or is making high-pitched noises, it is severe choking.

- Stand (or kneel for a small child) behind the person and wrap one arm diagonally across the person's chest.
- Bend the person forward at the waist until the person's upper airway is at least parallel to the ground.
- With the heel of your other hand, deliver five firm back blows between the shoulder blades.

> **NOTE:**
>
> To determine if choking is mild or severe, ask, "Are you choking?" If the person can speak, cough, or breathe, it is mild choking.

> **NOTE:**
>
> To deliver effective back blows, you may need to stand behind and slightly to the side of the person rather than directly behind the person.

3 If the object has not been dislodged, make a fist and place it just above the belly button.

- Place your other hand over the fist and pull sharply in and up, doing five abdominal thrusts.
- Continue the cycle of five firm back blows and five abdominal thrusts until the object comes out or the person begins to breathe or cough or becomes unconscious.

4 If the object comes out, perform a secondary survey and treat any non-life-threatening conditions.

5 Provide **continual care** and seek medical attention.

If the person becomes unconscious:

Support the person to the ground, protecting the head, and place the person on her back. Recheck the person's ABCs. Call EMS/9-1-1, get an AED, and follow the steps for unconscious, choking adult or child (see page 50).

 For a Larger or Pregnant Person

Alternate between five firm back blows and five **chest thrusts** when you cannot reach far enough around a person to perform **abdominal thrusts**, or if a woman is obviously pregnant. To perform chest thrusts:

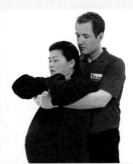

1. Stand behind the person and wrap both of your arms around the person's chest just under the armpits.

2. Make a fist and place the thumb side of the fist in the middle of the person's chest.

3. Place your other hand over your fist and pull straight back towards you. If the first couple of thrusts aren't effective, pull more sharply and deeply.

4. Continue alternating between five firm back blows and five chest thrusts until the object comes out or the person begins to breathe or cough or becomes unconscious.

 For Someone in a Seated Position

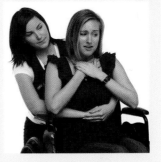

1. If the person is in a wheelchair, lock the wheels of the wheelchair.

2. Kneel or crouch behind the person.

3. Wrap both of your arms around the person's **abdomen**.

4. Make a fist with one hand and place the thumb side of the fist just above the person's belly button.

5. Grasp your fist with your other hand. Pull sharply in and up five times.

6. Make a fist with one hand and place the thumb side of the fist in the middle of the person's chest.

7. Place your other hand over your fist and pull straight back towards you sharply five times.

8. Continue alternating between abdominal thrusts and chest thrusts until the object comes out or the person begins to breathe or cough or becomes unconscious.

For Someone Choking Alone

1. Dial EMS/9-1-1 and leave the phone off the hook. This will tell the dispatcher to send help.

2. If there are people nearby, move to a place where you can get noticed.

3. Drop your abdomen onto a safe object with no sharp edges or corners, such as the back of a chair. Try to dislodge the object by doing thrusts on the same area you would use for abdominal thrusts.

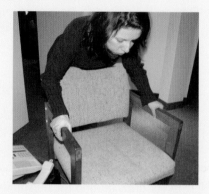

CONSCIOUS, CHOKING BABY

 What to Do

Check:

• Check the scene to ensure it is safe.

• If it is safe to do so, check the baby and the baby's ABCs.

Call:

• Shout for help.

Care:

• If a baby is coughing or gagging, the choking is mild. Do not interfere.

• If the baby is making high-pitched noises, is wheezing, can no longer make a sound, or becomes too weak to cough, have someone call EMS/9-1-1 and get an AED, then care for the baby:

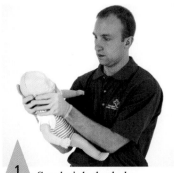

1 Sandwich the baby between your forearms, supporting the head.

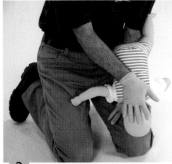

2 Turn the baby face down with the head lower than the body.

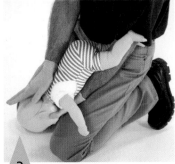

3 Lower your forearm onto your thigh. With the heel of your hand, deliver five firm back blows between the shoulder blades.

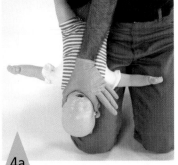

4a If the object has not been dislodged, while still supporting the head, turn the baby face up, with your arm supported on your thigh.

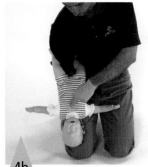

4b Place two fingers on the middle of the chest just below the nipple line and "push hard, push fast" at least 4 cm (1.5 in.) or $\frac{1}{3}$ to $\frac{1}{2}$ the depth of the chest five times.

4c Repeat the five firm back blows and five chest thrusts until the object is coughed up; the baby starts to cry, breathe, or cough; or the baby becomes unconscious.

5 If the object comes out or the baby starts to cry, breathe, or cough:

• Perform a secondary survey and treat any non-life-threatening conditions.

6 Provide continual care until EMS personnel arrive.

If the baby becomes unconscious, follow the steps for unconscious, choking baby (see page 52).

UNCONSCIOUS, CHOKING ADULT OR CHILD

 What to Do

Check:

- Check the scene to ensure it is safe.
- If it is safe to do so, check the person and the person's ABCs.

NOTE:
"Push hard, push fast." Compression depths: Adult—at least 5 cm (2 in.) Child—at least 5 cm (2 in.) or $^1/_3$ to $^1/_2$ the depth of the chest

Call:

- If the person does not respond, have someone call EMS/9-1-1 and get an AED.
- If you are alone with an adult, call EMS/9-1-1 yourself, get an AED, and then return to care for the person.
- If you are alone with a child, do five cycles (two minutes) of CPR first, then call EMS/9-1-1, get an AED, and return to care for the child.

Care:

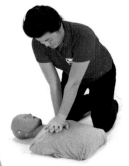 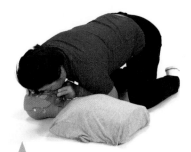 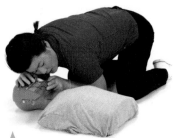

1 Start chest compressions:

- Place the heel of one hand on the middle of the person's chest. Place the other hand on top.
- Do 30 compressions. "Push hard, push fast."
- Allow the chest to recoil after each compression.

2a Give one rescue breath:

- Open the airway using the head-tilt/chin-lift.
- Pinch the person's nostrils closed.
- Take a normal breath.
- Cover the person's mouth with your mouth.
- Give one breath lasting one second, with just enough volume to make the chest start to rise.

2b If the person's chest does not rise after the first breath, perform the head-tilt/chin-lift again, tilting the head farther back and attempt to give another breath.

NOTE:
If there is any change in the person's condition during the CPR sequence, stop and check the person's ABCs.

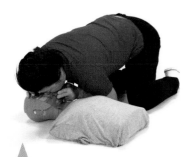

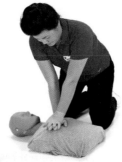

3a If your breath still does not go in, go to Step 4. If your first breath goes in, give a second breath.

3b When both breaths go in, and there is no obvious response to your two breaths, start the CPR sequence of 30 compressions and 2 breaths.

4 Repeat the cycle of 30 compressions, then look in the person's mouth.

• Grasp both the tongue and lower jaw and lift.

• If you do not see an object, return to Step 2a.

• If you can see an object, remove it. Turn the head to the side, slide your finger down the inside of the cheek to the base of the tongue, and try to sweep the object out. When the object is out of the person's mouth, return to Step 2a.

5 Continue CPR until:

• An AED arrives.

• More advanced care takes over.

• The scene becomes unsafe.

• You become physically unable to continue.

6 Provide continual care until EMS personnel arrive.

NOTE:
If your breath does not go in, go back to compressions.

NOTE:
After you reposition the head and attempt to give a second breath once, you do not need to repeat the repositioning step between chest compression cycles.

NOTE:
If there are two First Aiders present, they should alternate every five cycles (about two minutes).

NOTE:
CPR chest compressions should be done while the person is lying on a hard, flat surface.

NOTE:
It is important to minimize interruptions in chest compressions.

UNCONSCIOUS, CHOKING BABY

 What to Do

Check:

- Check the scene to ensure it is safe.
- If it is safe to do so, check the baby and the baby's ABCs.

Call:

- If the baby does not respond, have someone call EMS/9-1-1 and get an AED.
- If you are alone with the baby, do five cycles (two minutes) of CPR first. As long as you don't suspect a head and/or spine injury, take the baby with you to call EMS/9-1-1, get an AED, and then return to providing care.

Care:

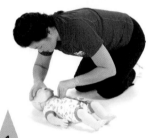

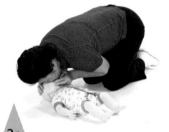

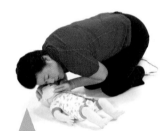

1 Start chest compressions:

- Place two fingers on the middle of the baby's chest, just below the nipple line.
- Do 30 compressions. "Push hard, push fast."
- Allow the chest to recoil after each compression.

2a Give one rescue breath:

- Open the airway using the head-tilt/chin-lift.
- Take a normal breath.
- Cover the baby's mouth and nose with your mouth.
- Give one breath lasting one second, with just enough volume to make the chest start to rise.

2b If the baby's chest does not rise after the first breath, perform the head-tilt/chin-lift again.

NOTE:
"Push hard, push fast." Compression depth: Baby—at least 4 cm (1.5 in.) or $^1/_3$ to $^1/_2$ the depth of the chest.

NOTE:
If there is any change in the baby's condition during the CPR sequence, stop and check the baby's ABCs.

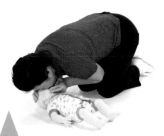 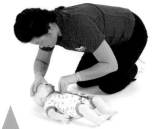

3a Attempt to give another breath. If your breath still does not go in, go to Step 4. If your first breath goes in, give a second breath.

3b When both breaths go in and there is no obvious response to your two breaths, start the CPR sequence of 30 compressions and 2 breaths.

 4 Repeat the cycle of 30 compressions, then look in the mouth.

• Grasp both the tongue and lower jaw and lift.

• If you do not see an object, return to Step 2a.

• If you can see an object, remove it. Turn the head to the side, slide your finger down the inside of the cheek to the base of the tongue, and try to sweep the object out. When it is removed, return to Step 2a.

 5 Continue CPR until:

• An AED arrives.

• More advanced care takes over.

• The scene becomes unsafe.

• You become physically unable to continue.

6 Provide continual care until EMS personnel arrive.

NOTES:

Breathing and Circulation Emergencies

Breathing and Circulation Emergencies

After a very fast-paced shift on the soccer field, a teenaged player cannot catch her breath. The condition gets worse very quickly, and she loses consciousness and collapses at the side of the field.

Breathing Emergencies

A person having difficulty breathing is in **respiratory distress**. A person who can't breathe at all is in **respiratory arrest**. Both respiratory distress and respiratory arrest are **breathing emergencies**. Brain **cells** begin to die in four to six minutes without oxygen (Figure 6.1).

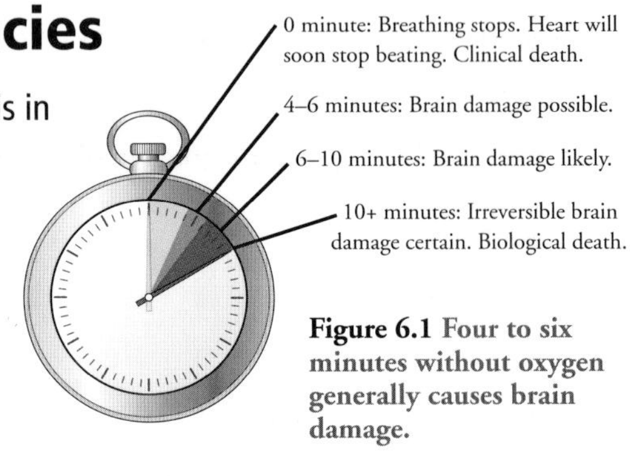

0 minute: Breathing stops. Heart will soon stop beating. Clinical death.

4–6 minutes: Brain damage possible.

6–10 minutes: Brain damage likely.

10+ minutes: Irreversible brain damage certain. Biological death.

Figure 6.1 Four to six minutes without oxygen generally causes brain damage.

RESPIRATORY DISTRESS

> #### Common Causes

- Hyperventilation
- Asthma
- **Allergic reaction** or anaphylaxis
- Chest injury

HYPERVENTILATION

Hyperventilation occurs when breathing is faster than normal. This upsets the body's balance of oxygen and carbon dioxide.

> #### Causes

- Emotion, such as excitement, fear, or anxiety
- Injuries to the head
- Severe bleeding
- Some medical conditions or illnesses

- Asthma
- Exercise
- Injury

Prevention

If you tend to hyperventilate due to anxiety, panic, or stress, practise breathing exercises or relaxation techniques.

If you hyperventilate due to an underlying medical condition, a doctor will help you understand and treat your condition.

 What to Look For

- Rapid, shallow breathing
- A feeling of suffocating or not getting enough air
- Fear, anxiety, or confusion
- Dizziness and numbness or tingling of the fingers and toes

 What to Do

Check:

- Check the scene to ensure it is safe.
- If it is safe to do so, check the person and the person's ABCs.

Call:

- Have someone call EMS/9-1-1 and get an AED if there are signs and symptoms of an injury or an underlying illness or condition, the hyperventilation does not stop after a few minutes, or the person becomes unconscious. If you are alone, call EMS/9-1-1 yourself, get an AED, and then return to care for the person.

Care:

1. Ensure the person's ABCs are present.
2. Tell the person to relax and breathe slowly. You can often stop hyperventilation by reassuring the person.
3. Perform a secondary survey and treat any non-life-threatening conditions.
4. Provide continual care until EMS personnel arrive.

Assisting With Medications

Guidelines for First Aiders Assisting With Medications

- The ill or injured person should be capable of **self-administration of medication**.

- The ill or injured person must be conscious and able to clearly express any risks involved with taking the medication under the present conditions.

- Assistance should be limited to preparing medications that can be given orally or with auto-injectors that First Aiders know and understand.

- The ill or injured person should take oral medication only if he or she can swallow. The person should also be certain that nothing will interfere or react negatively with the medication. The person should read and follow all label or medical instructions.

- All Five Rights of Medication must be met.

NOTE:
Over-the-counter medications won't have the person's name on them.

Five Rights of Medication

1. **Right person:** Make sure the person getting the medication is the one whose name is on the label of the medicine container.

2. **Right medication:** Read the label when you are getting the medication.

3. **Right amount:** Use an accurately marked measuring container (if applicable).

4. **Right time:** Give the medication at the right time.

5. **Right method:** Read the directions carefully.

ASTHMA

During an asthma attack, the air passages become narrower and breathing is difficult. **Asthma** is more common in children. It is usually controlled with medication.

 Prevention

If you have asthma:

- Know what causes an asthma attack and avoid it if possible. Asthma is commonly triggered by:

  ▶ Reactions to air quality (e.g., cigarette smoke), pollen, food, a drug, an insect sting, or some animals

  ▶ Temperature fluctuations, extreme humidity, and extreme dryness

> ► Colds and flus
>
> ► Emotional stress
>
> ► Physical activity
>
> • Always have your prescribed medication nearby in case of an attack.
>
> If your child has asthma:
>
> • Make sure that anyone who supervises your child knows about the asthma and how to help give medication if necessary.

 What to Look For

During an asthma attack, a person may:

- Wheeze when **exhaling**
- Gasp for air or seem unable to catch his or her breath
- Be upset
- Feel his or her chest tightening or feel tingling in the hands and feet

 What to Do

Check:

- Check the scene to ensure it is safe.
- If it is safe to do so, check the person and the person's ABCs.

Call:

- Have someone call EMS/9-1-1 and get an AED if the person is struggling to breathe or if the person is not responding to his or her medication. If you are alone, call EMS/9-1-1 yourself, get an AED, and then return to care for the person.

Care:

1. Move the person into a well-ventilated area, away from the environment if this is what caused the attack.
   - Help the person get into a comfortable position.
   - Calm the person to help slow down his or her breathing.
2. Help the person to take any prescribed medication for his or her condition.
3. Ensure the person's ABCs are present.
4. Perform a secondary survey and treat any non-life-threatening conditions.
5. Provide continual care.

▶ How to Assist in the Use of an Inhaler (Puffer) With a Spacer[1]

1. Make sure that you check the Five Rights of Medication before proceeding (see page 58).

2. Tell the person to shake the **inhaler** three or four times.

3. Help the person remove the cap from the inhaler. If the person uses a spacer and it has a cap, help the person remove it.

4. Tell the person to put the inhaler into the spacer, if applicable.

5. Tell the person to breathe out, away from the inhaler and spacer.

6. For a child, help bring the spacer or the inhaler to the child's mouth (Figure 6.2). Help to put the mouthpiece between the child's teeth, then tell the child to close his or her lips around it. For an adult, help bring the spacer or the inhaler to his or her mouth.

7. Tell the person to press the top of the inhaler once. If the person is unable to do this, you may do it instead if the person asks you to.

8. Tell the person to take one slow, full breath, hold it for as long as comfortable, up to 10 seconds, and then breathe out.

Figure 6.2 An inhaler with a spacer and mask.

> **NOTE:**
>
> Some spacers come in the form of a mask.

ALLERGIC REACTIONS

Allergic reactions are sensitivities to specific substances that can be absorbed through the skin, inhaled into the lungs, swallowed, or injected.

▶ Prevention

- If you have an allergy to food, read ingredient labels carefully, and when eating out, ask questions about what is in the food.

- Avoid triggers such as foods and medications that have caused any type of allergic reaction in the past.

- If you have a child who is allergic to certain foods, introduce one new food at a time so you can recognize an allergic reaction.

[1]Adapted from The Lung Association. *Get Help: How to use puffers, inhalers, and other devices.* Available at www.lung.ca/diseases-maladies/help-aide/devices-dispositifs/index_e.php (accessed March 2011).

What to Look For

- Rash, itching, or hives (raised, itchy areas of skin) (Figure 6.3)

- A feeling of tightness in the chest and throat

- Weakness, dizziness, or confusion

 What to Do

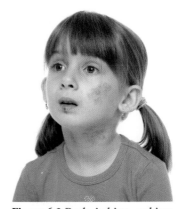

Figure 6.3 Rash, itching, or hives are a sign of an allergic reaction.

Check:

- Check the scene to ensure it is safe.

- If it is safe to do so, check the person and the person's ABCs.

Call:

- Have someone call EMS/9-1-1 and get an AED if the reaction is severe, if the person is struggling to breathe, or if the person loses consciousness. If you are alone, call EMS/9-1-1 yourself, get an AED, and then return to care for the person.

> **NOTE:**
>
> If the person develops an itchy rash, apply calamine lotion and cool compresses.

Care:

1. Ensure the person's ABCs are present.

2. Perform a secondary survey and treat any non-life-threatening conditions:

   - Calm and reassure the person having the reaction as anxiety can worsen symptoms.

   - Try to identify the allergen and have the person avoid further contact with it.

   - Watch the person for signs of increasing distress.

   - Provide continual care. Seek medical attention. For a mild reaction, the person's doctor may recommend over-the-counter medications (e.g., antihistamines).

ANAPHYLAXIS

Anaphylaxis is a severe allergic reaction. The air passages may swell, making breathing difficult. In some cases the person may go into respiratory arrest. Anaphylaxis may be caused by insect stings, food, medications, or other allergens.

 Prevention

- Be careful to avoid the substances, foods, or insects that cause a reaction.

- If you know that you have a severe allergy (anaphylaxis), wear a MedicAlert® medical identification product and carry your medication with you.

- Parents of a child with severe allergies must be especially vigilant and tell anyone looking after their child of the allergies and the possible reactions.

 What to Look For

LOOK OUT FOR...

Anaphylaxis can lead to death if it is not treated immediately.

The signs and symptoms of anaphylaxis may be similar to the signs and symptoms of an allergic reaction, but they are more pronounced:

- Swelling of the lips, face, neck, ears, and/or hands

- Generalized redness of the skin—this is often a raised, itchy, blotchy rash or hives

- Weakness or dizziness

- Nausea or vomiting

- Breathing difficulty, coughing, wheezing, or high-pitched noises. Tongue and throat swelling may block the airway

 What to Do

Check:

1. Check the scene to ensure it is safe.

2. If it is safe to do so, check the person and the person's ABCs.

Call:

- Have someone call EMS/9-1-1 and get an AED. If you are alone, call EMS/9-1-1 yourself, get an AED, then return to care for the person.

Care:

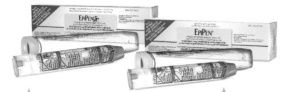

1 If the person has an **epinephrine** auto-injector, help the person use it.

2 Ensure the person's ABCs are present.

3 Perform a secondary survey and treat any non-life-threatening conditions:
- Calm the person to help slow down his or her breathing.
- Help the person get into a comfortable position.

4 Provide continual care until EMS personnel arrive.
- If conscious, the person may want to take additional medication such as an antihistamine.

> **NOTE:**
> Have the person check his or her pockets prior to using the auto-injector to ensure they don't contain anything that could block the auto-injector.

> **NOTE:**
> Ensure EMS/9-1-1 has been alerted anytime an auto-injector is being used.

▶ How to Assist in the Use of an Epinephrine Auto-Injector

1 Make sure that you check the Five Rights of Medication before proceeding (see page 58).

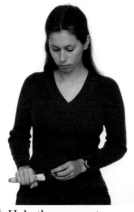

2 Help the person to remove the safety cap.

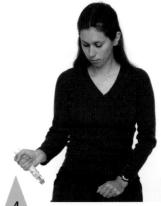

3 Tell the person to place the injection tip against her outer thigh and push the epinephrine auto-injector firmly against the thigh with a quick motion. A click should be heard. Hold for 10 seconds. If the person is unable to do this, you may do it instead if the person asks you to.

4 Have the person remove the epinephrine auto-injector.

5 Make sure the used epinephrine auto-injector goes with the person to the hospital.

RESPIRATORY ARREST

A person who stops breathing is in respiratory arrest. Without prompt first aid, respiratory distress can lead to respiratory arrest.

 Causes

- Suffocation
- Strangulation
- Airway obstruction
- Electrocution
- Drowning
- Drugs and alcohol
- Injury to the head, chest, or lungs
- A severe allergic reaction to food or an insect sting
- Respiratory conditions (e.g., emphysema or asthma)
- Poisoning, such as inhaling or swallowing something toxic

 What to Look For

- Unconsciousness
- Bluish lips and a face that is paler than normal
- Lack of movement in the chest and abdomen, except for the occasional attempt to breathe
- Lack of breathing sounds, except for the occasional gasp or gurgle

First aid for respiratory arrest is covered in Chapter 7 (and in Chapter 14 if you're a healthcare provider).

Circulation Emergencies

During coffee break at the warehouse where you work, one of the forklift drivers complains about pain in his chest. You notice that he is looking pale and is sweating.

 Prevention

Although a heart attack may seem to strike suddenly, cardiovascular disease develops over a long period of time. In fact, it can begin as early as the teenage years.

To prevent cardiovascular disease and heart attacks, you should follow the guidelines for a healthy lifestyle described below.

 Nutrition

A healthy lifestyle starts with a healthy, balanced diet. Each day you should have something from the four basic food groups: grain products, vegetables and fruits, milk and alternatives, and meat and alternatives. Check *Canada's Food Guide* to find out how much you should be eating from each food group.

Keep these points in mind as well:

- Fluids are important. Drink plenty of water each day. Eight 8-oz (236-mL) glasses each day are recommended.

- Fibre is important. Good sources include whole-grain breads and cereals, fruits, and leafy vegetables.

- Avoid foods that are high in salt, fat, and cholesterol (e.g., burgers, fries, etc.).

> **NOTE:**
>
> It is important to have some salt in your diet.

To improve your eating habits:

- Know the food you buy. Read the labels!

- Choose lower-fat substitutes for high-fat dairy products.

- Use non-hydrogenated oils and fats for cooking.

Weight Control

Having too much body fat can lead to heart disease, high blood pressure, diabetes, and gallbladder disease.

Losing weight, especially fat, is not easy. Your weight depends on the balance between how much you eat and how many calories you use through the day. However, other factors can also affect your weight, including thyroid problems, hormones, and when you eat.

To lose body fat:

- Get your body fat percentage checked by a certified trainer or doctor.
- Eat fewer calories than you use, but try to lose body fat gradually.
- Exercise regularly. Exercise is a key part of controlling your body fat.

 ## Exercise

Exercise is good for the heart, lungs, blood vessels, and muscles. Even if you don't have a lot of time for exercise, try to increase your cardiovascular fitness. This helps you:

- Cope with everyday stress
- Control your body fat
- Fight infections
- Improve your self-esteem
- Sleep better

Try to exercise at least three times a week for 20 to 30 minutes at your target heart rate. This rate is 65 to 85 percent of your maximum heart rate, which goes down as you get older. Talk to your doctor or fitness trainer to plan a proper training program.

Turn your daily activities into exercise. Look for ways to make exercise fun so that it is easier to make it a regular habit. If you have not been active, or if you have health problems, see your doctor before you start an exercise program.

 ## Stress Control

Stress is a normal part of life. If you learn how to cope with it well, you can help prevent illness and stay healthy. To reduce stress:

- Develop rewarding hobbies.
- Exercise regularly.
- Avoid coffee, tea, chocolate, soft drinks, or pain relievers that contain caffeine, which can reduce your ability to handle stress.
- Set goals that you can reach. Unrealistic goals will only add to your stress.
- Practise relaxation exercises. Sit or lie quietly in a comfortable position with your eyes closed. Breathe in deeply through your nose and out through your mouth. Focus on your breathing for 10 minutes.

Breaking Unhealthy Habits: Smoking

In the past few decades, the dangers of smoking have become well known. Smoking is banned or restricted in most work sites and public places.

Smoking tobacco is the most preventable cause of heart disease. Smoking also causes most cases of lung cancer, and it can lead to other forms of respiratory distress. Fortunately, the risk of respiratory and cardiovascular problems starts to drop as soon as you stop smoking.

Smokeless tobacco is also dangerous. Chewing tobacco and snuff cause cancer of the mouth, tongue, and nasal passages.

There are many programs available to help smokers break the habit. Contact your local public health unit for more information.

ANGINA

Angina is chest pain or pressure that comes and goes.

 Causes

- Cardiovascular disease

- Anemia

- Certain heart disorders

 What to Look For

The signs and symptoms of angina are similar to the signs and symptoms of a heart attack, but:

- The pain usually lasts less than 10 minutes.

- The pain usually goes away if the person rests.

- The pain is usually helped by the person's medication.

HEART ATTACK

A heart attack happens when the heart can't get enough oxygen because of a blockage in one of the arteries feeding the heart muscle (Figure 6.4). A heart attack is caused by cardiovascular disease. Cardiovascular disease is any disease that affects the heart or the blood vessels.

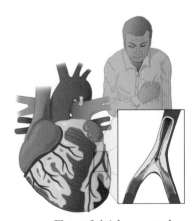

Figure 6.4 A heart attack.

Risk Factors for Developing Cardiovascular Disease

Controllable factors:

- Smoking
- Poor diet (especially a diet that is high in **cholesterol**)
- Stress
- High blood pressure
- Obesity
- Lack of regular exercise

Other factors:

- Gender
- **Heredity**
- Age

What to Look For

NOTE:
Not everyone experiences chest pain during a heart attack.

- Squeezing chest pain
- Problems breathing
- Abdominal or back pain (more common in women)
- Cold, sweaty skin
- Skin that is bluish or paler than normal
- Nausea and vomiting
- Denial
- Jaw pain

During a heart attack many women, elderly people, and people with **diabetes** tend to experience "soft signs," including:

- Mild, unfocused chest discomfort that:
  - ▶ Comes and goes
  - ▶ Doesn't feel like pain
  - ▶ Starts mild and gets continually stronger
  - ▶ Gets better with rest
  - ▶ Gets worse with activity

NOTE:
Men may have these signs as well.

- Tiredness
- Gastric discomfort
- Flu-like symptoms

ANGINA AND HEART ATTACK

 What to Do

Check:

- Check the scene to ensure it is safe.
- If it is safe to do so, check the person and the person's ABCs.

Call:

- Have someone call EMS/9-1-1 and get an AED. If you are alone, call EMS/9-1-1 yourself, get an AED, and then return to care for the person.

Care:

1. Have the person rest comfortably.
2. Assist the person in taking his or her medications such as ASA and nitroglycerin (if the person has it) after checking the Five Rights of Medication.
   - Nitroglycerin can come as a spray or pill. Nitroglycerin is sprayed or placed under the tongue.
3. Ensure the person's ABCs are present.
4. Perform a secondary survey and treat any non-life-threatening conditions.

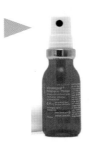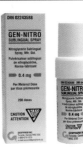

LOOK OUT FOR...

Erectile dysfunction drugs can cause a fatal lowering of blood pressure if given in conjunction with nitroglycerin. If the person has taken an erectile dysfunction drug, advise him or her not to take nitroglycerin.

If someone is unconscious, never put anything in his or her mouth.

5. Provide continual care until EMS personnel arrive.

NOTE:

If the person has asthma or an allergy to ASA, suggest that he or she not take ASA.

NOTE:

ASA won't make the pain go away, but it helps stop clotting in the arteries, thus reducing damage to the heart. Do not repeat the dosage. Medications such as acetaminophen (e.g., Tylenol®) or ibuprofen (e.g., Advil®) do not have the same effect as ASA in reducing damage due to heart attacks. Do not substitute!

TRANSIENT ISCHEMIC ATTACK (TIA)

A transient ischemic attack (TIA) is like a "mini-stroke," caused by a temporary drop in blood flow to part of the brain.

 ## Causes

- A clot in an artery in the brain
- An artery in the brain that ruptures
- A tumour

 ## What to Look For

The signs and symptoms of a TIA are the same as the signs and symptoms of a stroke (see page 71), but they disappear within a few minutes or hours.

 ## What to Do

Follow the same Check, Call, Care steps as for a stroke.

STROKE

A stroke happens when the blood flow to the brain gets interrupted (Figure 6.5).

 ## Causes

- A clot in an artery in the brain
- An artery in the brain that ruptures
- A tumour

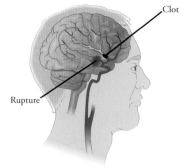

Clot

Rupture

Figure 6.5 A stroke can be caused by a clot or a rupture.

 ## Prevention

The risk factors for stroke are similar to those for heart disease. You can help prevent stroke with the same lifestyle changes discussed in the earlier section on preventing cardiovascular disease.

▶ **What to Look For**

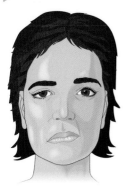

Figure 6.6 Facial numbness or weakness.

Remember FAST:

FACE—facial numbness or weakness, especially on one side (Figure 6.6)

ARM—arm numbness or weakness, especially on one side

SPEECH—slurred speech or difficulty speaking or understanding

TIME—time is important; call EMS/9-1-1 immediately

> **NOTE:**
>
> Other signs and symptoms of a stroke include:
> - a sudden, severe headache
> - dizziness or confusion
> - unconsciousness or temporary loss of consciousness
> - sudden loss of bladder control

 What to Do

Check:

- Check the scene to ensure it is safe.
- If it is safe to do so, check the person and the person's ABCs.

Call:

- Have someone call EMS/9-1-1 and get an AED. If you are alone, call EMS/9-1-1 yourself, get an AED, and then return to care for the person.

Care:

1. Ensure the person's ABCs are present.

2. Perform a secondary survey and treat any non-life-threatening conditions.

3. Have the person rest. Place the person in the recovery position with the affected side up, if possible. Reassure the person until EMS personnel arrive because this can be an extremely frightening experience.

DEADLY BLEEDING

Deadly bleeding is severe bleeding that leads to large amounts of blood loss, either outside or within the body. Deadly bleeding must be controlled immediately or it can become life-threatening.

 ## Causes

- An injury that breaks a blood vessel (an artery or **vein**)

 ## Prevention

- Be familiar with your surroundings.
- Keep all sharp objects, such as knives, in a safe place.
- Be aware of any machinery in the workplace.
- Wear appropriate safety equipment at work and at home.
- Be familiar with your equipment.
- Get proper training on machinery in the workplace.
- Stay alert.

EXTERNAL DEADLY BLEEDING

What to Look For

- Large amounts of bleeding (Figure 6.7)
- Signs of shock

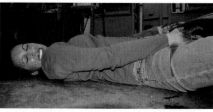

Figure 6.7 External deadly bleeding.

 ## What to Do

Check:

- Check the scene to ensure it is safe.
- If it is safe to do so, check the person and the person's ABCs.

Call:

- Have someone call EMS/9-1-1 and get an AED. If you are alone, call EMS/9-1-1 yourself, get an AED, then return to care for the person.

> **REMEMBER:**
> Wear personal protective equipment.

Care:

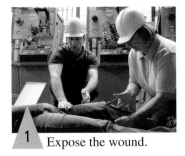

1. Expose the wound.

2. Apply direct pressure to the bleeding.

3. Secure the dressing.

4. Ensure the person's ABCs are present.

5. Perform a secondary survey and treat any non-life-threatening conditions.

6. Provide continual care until EMS personnel arrive.

INTERNAL DEADLY BLEEDING

▶ What to Look For

- Bruising in the injured area (Figure 6.8)
- **Soft tissues** (e.g., the abdomen) that are tender, swollen, or hard
- Shock
- Blood in saliva or vomit
- Pain
- Severe thirst
- Anxiety, nausea, and vomiting

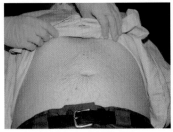

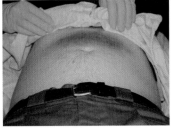

A   B

NOTE:

You should suspect internal bleeding in any injury that involved a forceful blow to the body.

Figure 6.8 Internal deadly bleeding. Before (A) and after (B).

Internal bleeding is more difficult to recognize than **external bleeding** because the signs and symptoms are less obvious and they may take longer to appear.

What to Do

Check:

- Check the scene to ensure it is safe.

- If it is safe to do so, check the person and the person's ABCs.

NOTE:

Remember your gloves
and other barrier devices.

Call:

- Have someone call EMS/9-1-1 and get an AED. If you are alone, call EMS/9-1-1 yourself, get an AED, then return to care for the person.

Care:

1. Help the person rest in the most comfortable position.

2. Ensure the person's ABCs are present.

3. Perform a secondary survey and treat any non-life-threatening conditions.

4. Provide continual care until EMS personnel arrive.

CARDIAC ARREST

Cardiac arrest occurs when the heart stops beating.

▶ Causes

Cardiovascular disease is the most common cause of cardiac arrest. Other common causes include:

- Drowning
- Suffocation
- Certain drugs
- Other heart diseases or abnormalities

- Severe blood loss
- Electrocution
- Severe chest injuries

▶ What to Look For

- Unconsciousness
- No signs of normal breathing

What to Do

Because the brain and other vital organs can live for only a few minutes after the heart stops beating, someone in cardiac arrest needs CPR, **defibrillation**, and advanced emergency medical care as soon as possible.

CPR combines rescue breaths and chest compressions to keep oxygen-rich blood circulating throughout the body. CPR will keep a minimal amount of blood moving to the vital organs until an AED is available and EMS personnel arrive.

An AED is a machine that analyzes the heart's electrical rhythm and, if necessary, tells the user to deliver a shock to the person in cardiac arrest. This is called defibrillation. The shock helps the heart re-establish an effective rhythm.

Studies show that if you can defibrillate someone quickly, the chance of survival increases greatly.

Public Access Defibrillation (PAD) is a movement to make AEDs readily available in many public areas, such as arenas or shopping centres. The advantage of AEDs is that it doesn't take intensive training to use them. With a little training and with voice prompts from the machine, users can successfully defibrillate someone in cardiac arrest. Contact your local city or municipality to find out if there is a PAD program in your area.

NOTES:

Respiratory and Cardiac Arrest

Respiratory and Cardiac Arrest

On the twelfth hole, your friend raises his club but never makes the swing. He collapses on the grass, unconscious. He doesn't seem to be breathing.

ROLLING A PERSON

If someone is face down and you cannot check if she is breathing in that position, you will need to roll the person over:

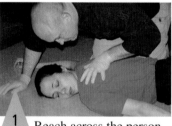

1 Reach across the person and grab any clothing close to the waist that is strong enough to pull on.

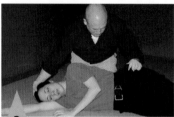

2 Try to support the head and neck while rolling the person to prevent the head from hitting the floor. Roll the person towards you.

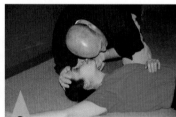

3 Once you have the person on her back, open the airway and check breathing.

COMPRESSION-ONLY CPR

Compression-only CPR uses chest compressions to pump the heart and circulate oxygen already in the person's body. Compression-only CPR is suitable when:

- An adult collapses suddenly.
- A bystander is unwilling, unable, or not sure how to perform full CPR, or is waiting for trained assistance to arrive.
- A responder does not have a breathing barrier (e.g., a mask) and does not want to perform unprotected rescue breaths.

Compression-only CPR should not be used when caring for:

- A drowning person
- A respiratory emergency that may have caused the cardiac arrest
- A child or baby

RESPIRATORY AND CARDIAC ARREST, ADULT OR CHILD

 What to Do

Check:

- Check the scene to ensure it is safe.
- If it is safe to do so, check the person and the person's ABCs.

Call:

- If the person does not respond, have someone call EMS/9-1-1 and get an AED.
- If you are alone with an adult, call EMS/9-1-1 yourself, get an AED, and then return to care for the person.
- If you are alone with a child, do five cycles (two minutes) of CPR first, then call EMS/9-1-1, get an AED, and return to care for the child.

Care:

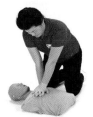 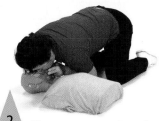 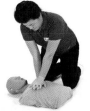

1 Start CPR:

- Place the heel of one hand on the middle of the person's chest. Place the other hand on top.
- Do 30 compressions. "Push hard, push fast."
- Allow the chest to recoil after each compression.

2 Give two rescue breaths:

- Open the airway using the head-tilt/chin-lift.
- Pinch the person's nostrils closed.
- Take a normal breath.
- Cover the person's mouth with your mouth.
- Give two breaths. Each breath should last one second, with just enough volume to make the chest start to rise.

3a If both breaths go in:

- Repeat the cycle of 30 compressions and 2 breaths.

3b If your breaths do not go in, follow the care steps for "Unconscious, Choking Adult or Child" in Chapter 5.

4 Continue CPR until:

- An AED arrives.
- More advanced care takes over.
- The scene becomes unsafe.
- You become physically unable to continue.

5 Provide continual care until EMS personnel arrive.

> **NOTE:**
> If there are two First Aiders present, they should alternate every five cycles (about two minutes).

> **NOTE:**
> "Push hard, push fast."
> Compression depths:
> Adult—at least 5 cm (2 in.)
> Child—at least 5 cm (2 in.) or $1/3$ to $1/2$ the depth of the chest

RESPIRATORY AND CARDIAC ARREST, BABY

 What to Do

Check:

- Check the scene to ensure it is safe.
- If it is safe to do so, check the baby and the baby's ABCs.

Call:

- If the baby does not respond, have someone call EMS/9-1-1 and get an AED.
- If you are alone with the baby, do five cycles (two minutes) of CPR first. As long as you don't suspect a head and/or spine injury, take the baby with you to call EMS/9-1-1 and get an AED and then return to providing care.

Care:

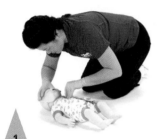

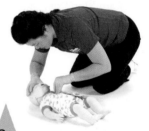

1 Start CPR:

- Keep the airway open by using your hand to maintain a head-tilt.
- Place two fingers on the middle of the chest, just below the nipple line.
- Do 30 compressions. "Push hard, push fast."
- Allow the chest to recoil after each compression.

2 Give two breaths with just enough volume to make the chest start to rise:

- Take a normal breath.
- Seal your lips tightly over the baby's mouth and nose.
- Give two breaths. Each breath should last one second, with just enough volume to make the chest start to rise.

3a If both breaths go in:

- Repeat the cycle of 30 compressions and 2 breaths.

3b If your breaths do not go in, follow the care steps for "Unconscious, Choking Baby" in Chapter 5.

NOTE:

"Push hard, push fast."

Compression depth:

Baby—at least 4 cm (1.5 in.) or $^1/_3$ to $^1/_2$ the depth of the chest

4 Continue CPR until:

- An AED arrives.
- More advanced care takes over.
- The scene becomes unsafe.
- You become physically unable to continue.

5 Provide continual care until EMS personnel arrive.

When the AED Arrives:

1. Open and turn on the AED.

2. Remove any clothing or objects (including jewellery) from the person that may come in contact with the pads. Remove any medical patches, including nitroglycerin, nicotine, or hormone, that you see. Use gloves so that you don't absorb the medication through your hands.

3. Ensure that the chest is dry and free of hair so the pads can stick. If the person has a lot of chest hair, shave it off using the razor included with the AED. If there is no razor, you can use an extra set of pads to remove the hair by sticking them on and then pulling them off the person's chest.

4. Follow the diagrams on the pads to place them on the person. Use the appropriate pad—adult, child, or baby—based on the person's age.

5. Check whether the person has an implanted pacemaker. Look on the chest for a small scar and a lump about the size of a matchbox. If the person has a pacemaker, apply the AED pads approximately 2.5 cm (1 in.) away from the pacemaker.

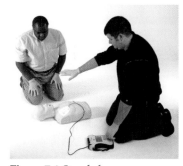

6. Follow the AED's automated prompts.

7. When the AED prompts you to give a shock (Figure 7.1), stand clear and say, "I'm clear, you're clear, everybody's clear." Make sure that no one is touching the person in cardiac arrest during the "analyze" and "shock" modes.

Figure 7.1 Stand clear.

A child is considered as being between one and eight years old. If child AED pads are unavailable, use adult pads. Follow the directions for pad placement.

A baby is considered as being one year old or less. If baby AED pads are unavailable, use child or adult pads. Follow the directions for pad placement.

If there is less than 2.5 cm (1 in.) between the pads when these are placed on the chest, place one on the front of the chest (anterior) and one on the back (posterior).

NOTE:

If the person is lying in a pool of water and/or blood, the "splash test" helps determine whether the person must be moved before using the AED. If you jump in the water and/or blood and there is a splash, the water and/or blood are deep enough to conduct electricity. The person must be removed from the water and/or blood before using the AED.

NOTE:

AED protocols can differ between jurisdictions. Ensure that you follow local protocol or the medical director's instructions, whichever is applicable in your area.

SPECIAL CONSIDERATIONS

▶ Air in the Stomach

Air in the stomach can make someone vomit. When an unconscious person vomits, the stomach contents may get into the lungs—a condition called aspiration. Aspiration makes giving rescue breaths more difficult, and it can reduce the person's chances of successful resuscitation. To prevent aspiration and the damage it can cause to lungs, give breaths only until the chest starts to rise.

▶ Vomiting

In some situations a person may vomit while you are giving CPR. If this happens:

1 Turn the person's head and body together as one unit onto the person's side, facing you.

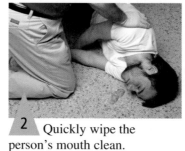 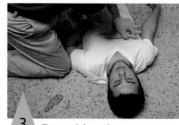

2 Quickly wipe the person's mouth clean.

3 Reposition the person on his back and continue with CPR.

▶ Mouth-to-Nose Breathing

Sometimes you cannot seal your mouth well over the person's mouth to give rescue breaths because:

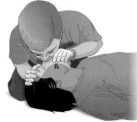

- The person's jaw or mouth is injured.
- The person's jaw or mouth is shut too tightly to open.
- Your mouth is too small to cover the person's mouth.
- The person has blood coming out of his or her mouth.

Figure 7.2 Mouth-to-nose breathing.

If this happens, breathe into the person's nose (Figure 7.2). Block the mouth to stop air from escaping.

▶ Mouth-to-Stoma Breathing

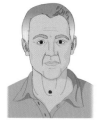

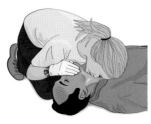

Some people have had an operation that removed part of their trachea. They breathe through an opening called a **stoma** in the front of the neck (Figure 7.3). Because air passes directly into the trachea through the stoma instead of through the mouth and nose, you should give rescue breaths into the stoma (Figure 7.4). Block the person's mouth and nose to stop air from escaping.

Figure 7.3 A stoma.   **Figure 7.4** Mouth-to-stoma breathing.

One-Hand Compressions

If you have arthritis or your hands aren't strong enough for regular compressions, the one-hand compression method may work:

1 Place the heel of one hand in the middle of the person's chest.

2 Grasp the wrist of the hand that is on the chest with your other hand.

3 Straighten your arms as much as possible without hurting yourself.

4 Begin compressions.

CPR for a Pregnant Woman

- If someone is available, ask the person to find a soft object that you can place under the woman's right hip (Figure 7.5).

- Raising the right hip 7.5 to 10 cm (3 to 4 in.) will help blood return to the heart. Do not interrupt CPR to find an object.

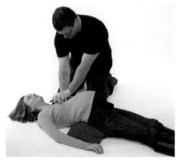

Figure 7.5 Place a soft object under the woman's right hip.

CPR SUMMARY

Adult	Child	Baby
Hand Position	**Hand Position**	**Hand Position**
Two hands on the middle of the chest	Two hands on the middle of the chest	Two fingers on the middle of the chest (just below the nipple line)
Compress	**Compress**	**Compress**
At least 5 cm (2 in.)	At least 5 cm (2 in.) or $1/3$ to $1/2$ of chest depth	At least 4 cm (1.5 in.) or $1/3$ to $1/2$ of chest depth
Breathe	**Breathe**	**Breathe**
Just enough volume to make the chest start to rise (1 second per breath)	Just enough volume to make the chest start to rise (1 second per breath)	Slowly, with just enough volume to make the chest start to rise (1 second per breath)
Cycle	**Cycle**	**Cycle**
30 compressions and 2 breaths	30 compressions and 2 breaths	30 compressions and 2 breaths
Compression Rate	**Compression Rate**	**Compression Rate**
30 compressions in about 18 seconds. Rate of at least 100 per minute (not including breathing)	30 compressions in about 18 seconds. Rate of at least 100 per minute (not including breathing)	30 compressions in about 18 seconds. Rate of at least 100 per minute (not including breathing)

Wound Care

Wound Care

On a camping trip, your four-year-old daughter trips and lands in the bright red embers of the campfire. You hear her crying and turn to see burns on the child's hands and arms, as well as a large splinter of wood sticking out of one hand.

Wounds such as bruises, scrapes, and small cuts are very common injuries. There are many ways to cause these types of wounds.

 Prevention

- Develop safe play habits to prevent injury, such as not running with sharp objects.

- Use helmets, knee pads, and elbow pads during sports and when using sports equipment such as bikes, skateboards, and in-line skates.

- Wear proper safety equipment in the workplace.

BRUISES

A bruise is a discoloured area of the skin that is created when blood and other fluids seep into nearby **tissues** (Figure 8.1).

 Causes

- Some kind of blow or impact to the body

 What to Look For

- Discolouring (red, purple, black, or blue areas)

- Swelling

- Pain

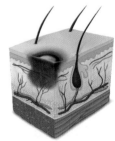

Figure 8.1 A bruise.

What to Do

Check:

- Check the scene to ensure it is safe.
- If it is safe to do so, check the person and the person's ABCs.

Call:

- Call EMS/9-1-1 if you suspect there may be more serious injuries.

Care:

1. Ensure the person's ABCs are present.
2. Perform a secondary survey and treat any non-life-threatening conditions:
   - Cool the area to help reduce pain and swelling.
   - When you cool the area, put some sort of cloth or pad between the ice and the skin.
   - Apply the ice for 20 minutes of every hour for as long as the person keeps feeling pain. Place a cloth between the ice and the person's skin.

> If a person feels severe pain or cannot move a body part without pain, or if you think the force that caused the injury was great enough to cause serious damage or severe bleeding, call EMS/9-1-1 and get an AED immediately. You may be dealing with internal bleeding, head and/or spine injuries, or bone, muscle, and **joint** injuries. See Chapters 6, 9, and 10 for instructions on how to care for these injuries.

CUTS AND SCRAPES

A cut is a wound where the skin has been split open or torn away. The edges of the wound can be jagged or smooth (Figure 8.2).

Scrapes are wounds where the skin has been rubbed or scraped away (Figure 8.3).

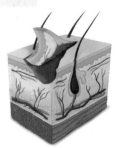

Figure 8.2 A cut.

 ### Causes

- Any action or sharp object that rubs or scrapes the skin away

What to Look For

- Possible bleeding
- Pain

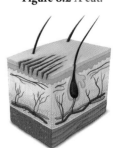

Figure 8.3 A scrape.

What to Do

Check:

- Check the scene to ensure it is safe.

- If it is safe to do so, check the person and the person's ABCs.

Call:

- Call EMS/9-1-1 and get an AED if you suspect that there may be more serious injuries.

NOTE:

Remember your gloves and other barrier devices.

Care:

- Ensure the person's ABCs are present.

- Perform a secondary survey and treat any non-life-threatening conditions:

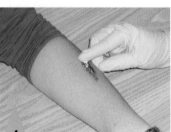

2 Wash the wound thoroughly with soap and water.

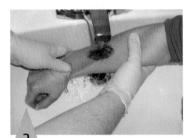

1 If gloves are not available, use some other kind of barrier between your hand and the wound. If possible, have the injured person use her own hand.

There is usually minimal bleeding with scrapes. If this is the case, go directly to Step 2. If there is bleeding, put direct pressure on the wound until it stops.

3 If possible, rinse the wound for five minutes with clean, running tap water.

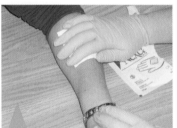

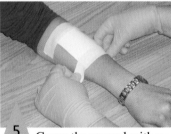

6 Watch for signs of infection. See "Infection" in this chapter.

4 If an antibiotic ointment or cream is available, put it on the wound as recommended by a pharmacist after checking the Five Rights of Medication. Ask the person if she has a sensitivity to any antibiotics, such as penicillin. If so, do not apply the ointment.

5 Cover the wound with a sterile non-stick dressing and/or bandage.

If there is a great deal of dirt or contamination in the wound, the injured person should seek medical attention.

If the blood soaks through the dressings, add more dressings on top. Do not remove the soaked dressings that are in direct contact with the wound! If you cannot control the bleeding, make sure the person gets medical attention immediately.

▶ A Stitch in Time

Wounds should be stitched by a trained medical professional in the first few hours after an injury. A wound may require stitching if:

- The edges of the skin do not fall together.
- The wound is more than 2.5 cm (1 in.) long.
- The wound is near joints on the hands or feet.
- The wound is on the face.

Stitches will help:

- Speed up healing
- Reduce the chance of infection
- Leave a less noticeable scar

PUNCTURE WOUNDS

A puncture wound happens when something pointed creates a hole in the skin (Figure 8.4).

▶ Causes

- Injuries from pointed objects such as nails or pieces of glass
- Animal bites

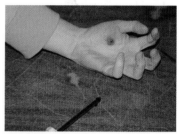

Figure 8.4 A puncture wound.

Prevention

- Develop safe play habits to prevent injury, such as not running with sharp objects.
- Wear proper safety equipment in the workplace and at home.
- Stay away from animals you are unfamiliar with.
- Wear shoes when walking outside.
- Always sweep up broken glass right away. Remove nails from boards and dispose of them properly.

 What to Look For

- Minimal external bleeding
- Possible bruising
- A hole where the object went through the skin

 What to Do

Check:

- Check the scene to ensure it is safe.
- If it is safe to do, check the person and the person's ABCs.

Call:

- Call EMS/9-1-1 and get an AED if the wound is deep or large.

Care:

- Ensure the person's ABCs are present.
- Perform a secondary survey and treat any non-life-threatening conditions:

NOTE:

Remember your gloves and other barrier devices.

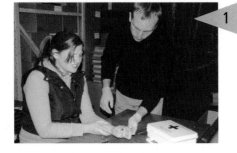

1 If gloves are not available, use some other kind of barrier between your hand and the wound. If possible, have the injured person use her own hand.

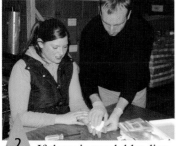

2 If there is much bleeding, put direct pressure on the wound until it stops.

3 Once the bleeding is controlled and there is no risk of causing more bleeding, wash the wound thoroughly with soap and water.

4 If possible, rinse the wound for five minutes with clean, running tap water.

5 If an antibiotic ointment or cream is available, put it on the wound as recommended by a pharmacist after checking the Five Rights of Medication. Ask the person if she has a sensitivity to any antibiotics, such as penicillin. If so, do not apply the ointment.

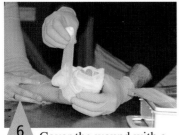

6 Cover the wound with a sterile dressing and/or bandage.

7 Watch for signs of infection over the next few days. See "Infection" in this chapter.

▶ Dressings and Bandages

Dressings are pads you put on an open wound to absorb blood and other fluids and to prevent infection. **Bandages** are materials you can use to wrap or cover a dressing. They are used to control bleeding, to apply pressure, to provide support, or to protect a wound from dirt and infection.

If a bandage is put on too tightly, the limb below the bandage may become cold or numb or begin to turn blue or paler than normal. If this happens, loosen the bandage.

If blood soaks through the bandage, use more dressings and another bandage. The dressing in contact with the wound should remain in place.

IMPALED OBJECTS

If the object that created the injury is stuck in the wound, it's called an **impaled object** (Figure 8.5).

 Causes

- Any force that causes an object to penetrate the skin and underlying tissues.

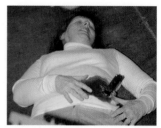

Figure 8.5 An impaled object.

 Prevention

- See "Puncture Wounds" in this chapter.

 What to Look For

- An object sticking out of the body
- Pain
- Shock
- Bleeding

What to Do

Check:

- Check the scene to ensure it is safe.
- If it is safe to do so, check the person and the person's ABCs.

LOOK OUT FOR:

If the impaled object is a weapon, ensure that the scene is safe.

Call:

- Call EMS/9-1-1 and get an AED if the impaled object is large or if it is impaled in the head, neck, or torso.

Care:

- Ensure the person's ABCs are present.
- Perform a secondary survey and treat any non-life-threatening conditions:

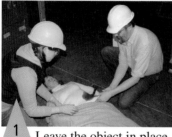

1 Leave the object in place.

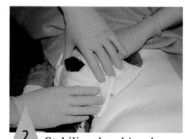

2 Stabilize the object by putting bulky dressings around it.

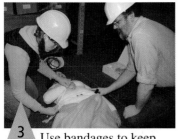

 3 Use bandages to keep the dressings in place.

4 Make sure the person gets medical attention.

NOSEBLEEDS

 ## Causes

- Forceful nose blowing
- Trauma to the nose
- High blood pressure
- Bleeding disorders
- Dry weather conditions

 ### Prevention

- Use a humidifier if the air indoors is dry.
- Wear protective athletic equipment when participating in sports that could cause injury to the nose.
- Encourage gentle nose blowing.

What to Look For

- Blood coming from the nose

 ### What to Do

Check:

- Check the scene to ensure it is safe.
- If it is safe to do so, check the person and the person's ABCs.

Call:

- Call EMS/9-1-1 and get an AED if the person loses consciousness, if the bleeding continues after 15 minutes, if the bleeding starts again, or if the bleeding was caused as a result of a medical condition or head injury.

Care:

- Ensure the person's ABCs are present.
- Perform a secondary survey and treat any non-life-threatening conditions:

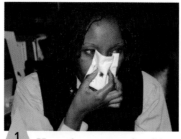

 Have the person sit with the head slightly forward while pinching the nostrils for 10 to 15 minutes.

2 Once you have controlled the bleeding, tell the person to avoid rubbing, blowing, or picking the nose because this could start the bleeding again.

3 If the person loses consciousness, place her in the recovery position to allow blood to drain from the nose.

 4 If the bleed was caused by an object in the nose and the object is easy to grasp, then gently pull it out. However, don't feel around inside the nostril with your finger. If there is an object in the nose that you cannot remove easily, the person should seek medical attention.

5 If the nosebleed was caused by a severe head injury, do not pinch the nose.

6 Provide continual care.

NOTE:
Remember your gloves and other barrier devices.

KNOCKED-OUT TEETH

▶ Causes

- Any kind of blow or fall that involves the mouth

▶ Prevention

- Wear appropriate equipment when playing sports, such as a mouthguard or face mask.
- Always wear a seat belt while in the car and do not eat or drink in a moving car.

▶ What to Look For

- Missing tooth, usually from some kind of impact
- Bleeding (although this is often very minimal)
- Pain in the mouth

What to Do

Check:

- Check the scene to ensure it is safe.
- If it is safe to do so, check the person and the person's ABCs.

Call:

- Call EMS/9-1-1 and get an AED if the knocked-out tooth was caused by a forceful blow to the head, the person was knocked unconscious, or you suspect that there may be other more serious injuries.

> Because a knocked-out tooth is often caused by an impact, the person may also have airway problems (see Chapter 5) or head and/or spine injuries (see Chapter 9).

Care:

- Ensure the person's ABCs are present.
- Perform a secondary survey and treat any non-life-threatening conditions:

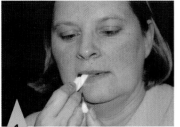

1 Control any bleeding by having the person bite down on a sterile or clean dressing.

2 Carefully pick up the tooth by the crown (the white part), not the root.

3 Gently rinse off the tooth in water. Do not scrub it or remove any tissue fragments that are attached.

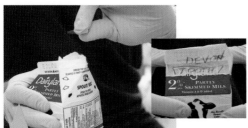

4 Put the tooth in milk, if available, or in water and keep it with the person. If there is no milk or water, wrap the tooth in a clean cloth or gauze with some of the person's own saliva. Seal the container with tape and label it with the name of the person, date, and time.

5 Get the person to a dentist as soon as possible. The greatest chance for repair is during the first hour after the tooth was knocked out.

6 Provide continual care.

EYE INJURIES

 ## Causes

- Foreign objects or particles in the eye
- Impact to the eye
- Radiation or burns

 ### Prevention

- Wear appropriate equipment in the workplace (e.g., a hard hat, ear plugs, or safety glasses/face shields).
- Wear appropriate equipment when you are playing sports (e.g., wear a batting helmet when you are playing baseball.)
- Get trained on all equipment at your workplace that might be dangerous.

 ### What to Look For

- Pain and irritation in the eye
- Difficulty opening the eye
- Watering of the eye
- Redness
- Problems seeing properly
- Deformities

 ### What to Do

Check:

- Check the scene to ensure it is safe.
- If it is safe to do so, check the person and the person's ABCs.

Call:

- Call EMS/9-1-1 and get an AED if you suspect that there may be a head and/or spine injury, if there is an impaled object in or near the eye, or if the eye is out of the socket.

Care:

- Ensure the person's ABCs are present.
- Perform a secondary survey and treat any non-life-threatening conditons:

Injuries to the eyeball are very serious and require special care. Never put **direct pressure** on the eyeball.

If there is a **foreign object** in the eye but it is not impaled:

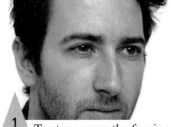

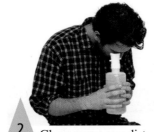

3 If the object remains in the eye, the person should seek medical attention.

1 Try to remove the foreign object by having the person blink several times. The eye will produce tears that may wash it out.

2 Clean away any dirt around the eye and then gently flush the eye with water (away from the unaffected eye).

If there is an impaled object in the eye:

1 Have the person rest comfortably.

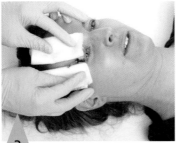

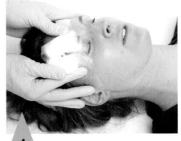

2 Leave the impaled object in the eye.

3 Stabilize the object by putting bulky dressings around it and being careful not to put pressure on the eye.

4 Use bandages to keep the dressings in place.

Flash burn

If the eyes were flash burned (e.g., from welding):

1. Cover the eyes with a cool, wet cloth.
2. Make sure the person gets medical attention.

Any wound near the eye should be treated as an eye injury.

EAR INJURIES

 ## Causes

- Impact
- Head injury
- Foreign objects or substances in the ear
- Cuts or tears
- Loud noise

 ## Prevention

- Wear proper protection when using loud equipment such as lawn mowers and chainsaws.

 ## What to Look For

- Blood or other fluid from within the ear
- Sudden or intense pain in the ear
- Hearing problems
- Swelling or deformity

What to Do

Check:

- Check the scene to ensure it is safe.
- If it is safe to do so, check the person and the person's ABCs.

Call:

- Call EMS/9-1-1 and get an AED if there is blood or other fluid draining from the ear.

If the ear injury is the result of an explosion or a diving injury, call EMS/9-1-1.

Care:

1. Ensure the person's ABCs are present.
2. Perform a secondary survey and treat any non-life-threatening conditions:
   - If the bleeding is from an external wound, treat it the same way you would treat any other wound.

If there is a foreign object in the ear, you don't suspect a head and/or spine injury, and the object looks like it can easily be removed:

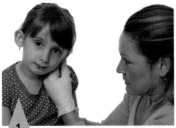

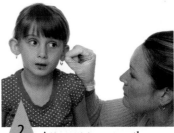

1 If you can see the object, remove it by tilting the head to the affected side. Then gently tap above the ear to loosen the object.

2 Attempt to grasp the object and pull it out.

If the person has a serious head and/or spine injury and blood or other fluid is in the ear canal or draining from the ear:

1. Let the ear drain. Do not apply direct pressure. Do not move the person if possible.

2. Cover the ear lightly with a sterile dressing.

3. Provide continual care until EMS personnel arrive.

NOTE:

Remember your gloves and other barrier devices.

INFECTION

An infection is a condition caused by the invasion of the body by germs (Figure 8.6).

 Causes

- Dirt, foreign bodies, or other things containing germs that get in a wound

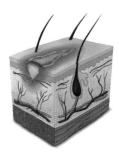

Figure 8.6 An infection.

 Prevention

- Always wash your hands before and after giving first aid.

- Whenever possible, wear gloves if you will be coming in contact with someone's body fluids.

- Whenever possible, use sterile dressings when you are caring for wounds.

- Keep your immunizations up to date. If you have been wounded and have not received a tetanus shot in more than five years, seek medical attention.

- Use antibiotic ointment on a wound to help reduce the risk of infection.

- Keep the wound area clean and wash regularly.

What to Look For

- Redness
- Pus
- Tenderness
- Swelling

- Red streaks moving away from the wound
- Heat or warmth
- Fever
- Nausea

AMPUTATIONS

An amputation is a complete or partial severing of a body part (Figure 8.7). Although there is a lot of damage to the tissues, bleeding is usually not severe.

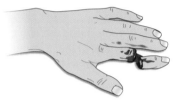

Figure 8.7 An amputation.

 Causes

- Any force great enough to completely or partially cut or tear away a limb or body part from the rest of the body

 Prevention

- Wear proper equipment when working around machinery.
- Follow the manufacturer's instructions when you are using equipment in the workplace or in the home.

 What to Look For

- Shock
- Pain
- A part of the body completely or partially disconnected from the rest of the body
- Bleeding

 What to Do

Check:

- Check the scene to ensure it is safe.
- If it is safe to do so, check the person and the person's ABCs.

Call:

- Have someone call EMS/9-1-1 and get an AED. If you are alone, call EMS/9-1-1 yourself, get an AED, and then return to care for the person.

Care:

- Ensure the person's ABCs are present.

- Perform a secondary survey and treat any non-life-threatening conditions:

1 Treat any bleeding with direct pressure.

2 Try to retrieve the amputated body part.

3 Wrap the amputated part in a clean cloth or gauze.

4 Place the amputated part in a plastic bag.

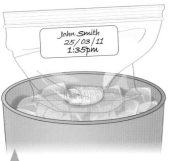

6 Label the container that contains the body part (person's name, date, and time).

7 Make sure the amputated part goes with the injured person to the hospital.

8 Provide continual care until EMS personnel arrive.

5 Keep the amputated part cool by placing the bag on ice and wrap it so that the body part does not freeze.

> **NOTE:**
>
> If the limb is partially disconnected from the body, put the limb back in place and treat the injury as an open wound or fracture.

CRUSH INJURIES

A **crush injury** occurs when there is a great deal of pressure on a part of the body.

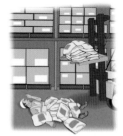

Figure 8.8 A crush injury.

 ## Causes

It is often caused by being squeezed between two heavy or immobile objects (Figure 8.8).

 ## Prevention

- Be familiar with your surroundings.
- Be familiar with your equipment and get trained in its proper use.
- Make sure your equipment is in good, safe, working order.
- Wear protective gear.
- Stay alert.

 ## What to Look For

- Person may still be crushed under the object(s) or between two objects
- Possible wound
- Deformity
- Signs of internal bleeding
- Shock
- Pain

NOTE:

Remove the object only if you can do it safely, without causing any further harm.

NOTE:

If the object is crushing the person's head, neck, chest, or abdomen, or the person cannot breathe, remove it immediately. If it is crushing another body part, leave the object where it is until EMS personnel arrive.

 ## What to Do

Check:

- Check the scene to ensure it is safe.
- If it is safe to do so, check the person and the person's ABCs.

Call:

- Have someone call EMS/9-1-1 and get an AED. If you are alone, call EMS/9-1-1 yourself, get an AED, and then return to care for the person.

Care:

1. Ensure the person's ABCs are present.
2. Perform a secondary survey and treat any non-life-threatening conditions.
3. Provide continual care until EMS personnel arrive.

PENETRATING CHEST INJURIES

Chest injuries can cause a breathing emergency if the lungs are punctured by a penetrating object. A puncture that goes through the rib cage may let air or blood into the chest through the wound (Figure 8.9).

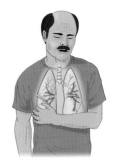

Figure 8.9 A penetrating chest injury.

Causes

- Weapons, such as knives or guns
- Falls onto objects
- Industrial incidents
- Other penetrating forces that create a wound in the chest wall

Prevention

Chest injuries can often be prevented by good safety practices in all areas of life, including:

- Driving motor vehicles
- Participating in sports and recreational activities
- Working around the home
- Performing occupational activities

Follow the safety guidelines throughout this manual for preventing injuries.

What to Look For

- Difficulty breathing
- Bleeding from an open chest wound (Figure 8.10)
- A sucking sound coming from the wound with each breath
- Severe pain at the site of the injury
- Coughing up blood
- Blood bubbling from the wound
- Gasping

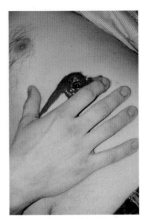

Figure 8.10 A bleeding, open chest wound.

What to Do

Check:

- Check the scene to ensure it is safe.
- If it is safe to do so, check the person and the person's ABCs.

Call:

- Have someone call EMS/9-1-1 and get an AED. If you are alone, call EMS/9-1-1 yourself, get an AED, and then return to care for the person.

Care:

- Ensure the person's ABCs are present.
- Perform a secondary survey and treat any non-life-threatening conditions:

NOTE:

Remember your gloves and other barrier devices.

---

1 Have the person rest in a comfortable position.

2 Cover the wound with a dressing that will stop air from getting into the chest, such as a piece of plastic wrap or a plastic bag.

3 Tape the dressing in place but leave the side closest to the ground open to allow for drainage. This method stops air from going into the chest cavity through the wound when the person breathes in but lets air escape when the person breathes out.

4 If breathing becomes difficult after applying the dressing, you may have to raise the open side to let trapped air escape.

5 Provide continual care until EMS personnel arrive.

PNEUMOTHORAX AND HEMOTHORAX

Chest injuries can lead to two conditions that can make breathing difficult: **pneumothorax** and **hemothorax** (Figure 8.11).

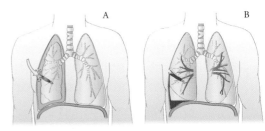

Figure 8.11 Pneumothorax (A) and hemothorax (B).

Causes

Pneumothorax is a condition in which air enters the chest cavity from the wound site but doesn't enter the lung. The air in the chest cavity presses against the lung, causing it to collapse.

Hemothorax is a condition in which blood accumulates in the chest cavity from the wound site but doesn't get into the lung. Because blood takes up space in the chest cavity, the lung can't expand effectively.

Prevention

See the prevention of penetrating chest injuries.

What to Look For

See what to look for with penetrating chest injuries.

What to Do

Follow the same Check, Call, Care steps as for penetrating chest injuries.

BLUNT CHEST INJURIES

Blunt chest injuries are caused by a direct blow to the chest, but they do not result in a hole in the chest wall (Figure 8.12).

Causes

- Motor vehicle collisions
- Falls
- Sports injuries
- Other crushing forces that do not create a wound in the chest wall

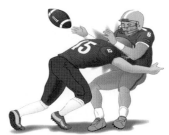

Figure 8.12 A blunt chest injury.

Prevention

See the prevention of penetrating chest injuries in this chapter.

What to Look For

- Pain
- Deformity or swelling
- Bruising at the site
- Shock
- Guarded, shallow breathing

 ## What to Do

Check:

- Check the scene to ensure it is safe.
- If it is safe to do so, check the person and the person's ABCs.

Call:

- Have someone call EMS/9-1-1 and get an AED. If you are alone, call EMS/9-1-1 yourself, get an AED, and then return to care for the person.

Care:

1. Ensure the person's ABCs are present.
2. Perform a secondary survey and treat any non-life-threatening conditions:
   - Keep the head and spine as still as possible as a blow to the chest may have caused head and/or spine injuries.
3. Provide continual care until EMS personnel arrive.

FLAIL CHEST

Flail chest is a condition in which the chest wall becomes unstable (Figure 8.13).

Causes

- Fractures of the breastbone
- Fractures of the cartilage connecting the ribs to the breastbone
- Fractures of the ribs

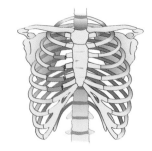

Figure 8.13 Flail chest.

What to Look For

- Difficulty breathing
- Painful breathing
- Crunching or grinding sounds in the chest
- Uneven rising of the chest during breathing
- Bruising on the chest
- Deformity or swelling
- Shock

What to Do

Check:

- Check the scene to ensure it is safe.
- If it is safe to do so, check the person and the person's ABCs.

Call:

- Have someone call EMS/9-1-1 and get an AED. If you are alone, call EMS/9-1-1 yourself, get an AED, and then return to care for the person.

Care:

1. Ensure the person's ABCs are present.
2. Perform a secondary survey and treat any non-life-threatening conditions:
   - Treat this injury as a blunt chest injury.
   - To help the person breathe better, give the person something bulky (such as a towel) to hold against the chest.
   - Keep the person still in case there are broken ribs.
3. Provide continual care until EMS personnel arrive.

BURNS

Burns are soft-tissue injuries caused by chemicals, electricity, heat, or radiation.

Prevention

Chemical burns

- Store chemicals in their original containers.
- Wear protective gear when you are handling chemicals.
- Wash your hands after touching chemicals.

- Get trained in the Workplace Hazardous Materials Information System (WHMIS), which will be changing to the Globally Harmonized System (GHS) of Classification and Labelling of Chemicals.

- Follow WHMIS, Material Safety Data Sheets (MSDS), and first aid labels on packages.

- Read the label before you use a product.

Electrical burns

- Keep electrical appliances away from water.

- If an electrical cord is frayed, fix it or get rid of it.

- If you have young children, cover electrical outlets.

Burns from lightning strikes

- As soon as you see or hear a storm, stop swimming or boating and get away from the water because water conducts electricity.

- Go inside the closest building. If there is no building nearby, get inside a car and roll up the windows.

- Stay away from the telephone, except in an emergency. If you are caught outside, stay away from telephone poles and tall trees.

- Stay off hilltops and try to crouch down in a ravine or valley if shelters are not available nearby.

- Stay away from farm equipment and small metal vehicles such as motorcycles, bicycles, and golf carts.

- Stay away from wire fences, clotheslines, metal pipes and rails, and other things that conduct electricity.

- If you are with a group of people, stay several metres apart from each other.

Thermal burns

- Keep matches away from children.

- Store gasoline and other highly flammable liquids outdoors.

- When you are cooking on the stove, turn the pot handles in and use only the back burners when possible.

- Keep the hot water tank temperature turned down to 49°C (120°F).

- Do not put water on a grease fire.

- Keep aerosol cans away from heat and open flames.

- Make sure your fireplace has a sturdy metal screen. Keep flammable materials away from fireplaces.

Sunburns

- Stay out of the sun between 10:00 a.m. and 3:00 p.m., if possible.

- Wear proper clothing to protect you from too much sun.

- Use a broad-spectrum sunscreen with a sun protection factor (SPF) of at least 30 and apply it 15 to 30 minutes before going outdoors. Reapply sunscreen at least every two hours, and after being in the water, or after vigorous activity and sweating.

▶ Fire safety

Fires are caused by many things: heating equipment, appliances, electrical wiring, and cooking.

Make sure you have working smoke detectors in the hallway near any sleeping areas, at the top of stairs, and in every bedroom. In some provinces and territories, legislation dictates where smoke detectors must be located.

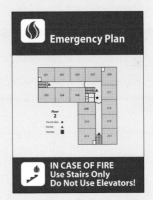

Plan and practise a fire escape route with your family:

- Sketch a floor plan of your home that shows all the rooms, doors, windows, and hallways.

- Draw arrows that show how to escape from each room. If possible, show two ways to get out of each room. Planning to escape sleeping areas is most important because most fires happen at night.

- Plan where everyone will meet after leaving the building.

- Assign someone to call the fire department after leaving the burning building.

- When you travel, take a moment to find out the local emergency number and keep it on hand.

- If you stay in a hotel, learn escape routes and emergency procedures in case of a fire.

To escape from a fire:

- If there is smoke, crawl to get out of the building.

- Make sure children can open windows, go down a ladder, or lower themselves to the ground. Practise with them.

- Get out quickly and never return to a burning building.

- If you cannot get out, stay in the room. Stuff towels, rags, or clothing around doors and vents. If you have access to water, wet these materials first. If there is a phone, call EMS/9-1-1, even if rescuers are already outside, and tell the dispatcher exactly where you are.

 What to Do

Check:

- Check the scene to ensure it is safe.

Call:

Call EMS/9-1-1 and get an AED immediately if:

- Burns make it hard for the person to breathe.
- The person is in a great deal of pain or becomes unconscious.
- Burns cover more than 10 percent of the person's body.
- Burns result from chemicals, explosions, or electricity.

Care:

- Follow the Check, Call, Care steps in Table 8.1.

Table 8.1 First Aid by Type of Burn

Types	Causes	What to Do

Chemical burns	Wet or dry chemicals	**Check:**
		• Check the scene to ensure it is safe.
		• If it is safe to do so, check the person and the person's ABCs.
		
		Call:
		• Have someone call EMS/9-1-1 and get an AED if the burn covers more than 10% of the body. If you are alone, call EMS/9-1-1 yourself, get an AED, and then return to care for the person.
		
		Care:
		1. Ensure the person's ABCs are present.
		2. Perform a secondary survey and treat any non-life-threatening conditions:
		  • Protect yourself by wearing protective equipment.
		  • Flush the affected areas with large amounts of cool running water for at least 15 minutes. Flush the chemicals away from areas of the body that have not been contaminated.
		  • Have the person remove any contaminated clothing.
		3. Seek medical attention.
		4. Refer to the appropriate MSDS or call your local Poison Control Centre for first aid measures.

> **NOTE:**
>
> If the chemical is dry, brush it off the skin carefully.

Types	Causes	🧰 What to Do

Electrical burns	Electricity
	Lightning
		Check:
		• Check the scene to ensure it is safe.
		• Make sure that trained personnel turn off the electrical current before you approach the person.
		• If it is safe to do so, check the person and the person's ABCs.
		
		Call:
		• Have someone call EMS/9-1-1 and get an AED. If you are alone, call EMS/9-1-1 yourself, get an AED, and then return to care for the person.
		
		Care:
		1. Ensure the person's ABCs are present. Electricity and lightning may affect the heart, so monitor the ABCs closely.
		2. Perform a secondary survey and treat any non-life-threatening conditions:
		  • Treat the person as if he or she might have a head and/or spine injury.
		  • Look for two burns (the entry and exit points). They will be open wounds that may need to be treated.
		3. Provide continual care until EMS personnel arrive.

Thermal burns	Liquid Steam Heat Flame	Cool the burn and treat according to the level of burn (see Table 8.2).
Radiation burns	Radioactive material	Refer to WHMIS.

Table 8.2 Seriousness of Burns

Level of Burn	What to Look For	What to Do
Superficial burns	Redness Pain Possible swelling 	**Check:** • Check the scene to ensure it is safe. • If it is safe to do so, check the person and the person's ABCs. **Call:** • You should not need to call EMS/9-1-1 for a superficial burn, unless the person is in a great deal of pain or becomes unconscious. **Care:** 1. Ensure the person's ABCs are present. 2. Perform a secondary survey and treat any non-life-threatening conditions: • Cool the burn with running or standing water for at least 10 to 20 minutes. If the standing water becomes warm, add more cool water. 3. Provide continual care. 4. Once the burning has stopped, you can apply an antibiotic ointment, after checking the Five Rights of Medication, and watch for infection. Your pharmacist or doctor can suggest products for superficial burns such as sunburns.

Level of Burn	What to Look For	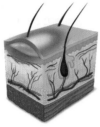 What to Do

Partial-thickness burns	Redness
	Pain
	Possible swelling
	Blisters
		Check:
		• Check the scene to ensure it is safe.
		• If it is safe to do so, check the person and the person's ABCs.
		Call:
		• Call EMS/9-1-1 and get an AED if the burn covers more than 10% of the body, the person is in a great deal of pain, or the person becomes unconscious.
		Care:
		1. Ensure the person's ABCs are present.
		2. Perform a secondary survey and treat any non-life-threatening conditions:
		  • If the burned area covers more than 10% of the person's body, call EMS/9-1-1, get an AED, and treat the person for shock. Cool only a small area at a time. Cooling the person too quickly may cause the person to go into shock.
		  • If the burned area covers less than 10% of the person's body, cool the burn with running or standing water for at least 10 to 20 minutes. If this is too painful or the area cannot be put in water, cover the burn with a cool, moist, sterile dressing or clean cloth to cool it.
		  • Only remove clothing around the affected area that is *not* stuck to the skin.
		  • After cooling the burn, cover it loosely with a dry, sterile dressing, preferably non-stick gauze.
		3. Seek medical attention.

NOTE:

A person's palm is approximately 1% of his or her body. This is a quick guide to calculate the percentage of the body burned.

Level of Burn	What to Look For	➕ What to Do

Full-thickness burns	Redness
	
	Pain (may not be present at the worst part of burn due to **nerve** damage)
	
	Possible swelling
	
	Blisters
	
	Charred or waxy, white flesh
	
	Open wound
		Check:
		• Check the scene to ensure it is safe.
		• If it is safe to do so, check the person and the person's ABCs.
		
		Call:
		• Have someone call EMS/9-1-1 and get an AED. If you are alone, call EMS/9-1-1 yourself, get an AED, and then return to care for the person.
		
		Care:
		1. Ensure the person's ABCs are present.
		2. Perform a secondary survey and treat any non-life-threatening conditions:
		  • If the burned area covers more than 10% of the person's body, call EMS/9-1-1, get an AED, and treat the person for shock. Cool only a small area at a time. Cooling the person too quickly may cause the person to go into shock.
		  • If the burned area covers less than 10% of the person's body, cool the burn with standing water. If this is too painful or the area cannot be put in water, cover the burn with a cool, moist, sterile dressing or clean cloth to cool it.
		  • Only remove clothing around the affected area that is *not* stuck to the skin.
		  • Do not try to clean a full-thickness burn.
		  • After cooling the burn, cover it loosely with a dry, sterile dressing, preferably non-stick gauze.
		3. Provide continual care until EMS personnel arrive.
		4. Have the person lie down and treat him or her for shock.

Special Considerations For Burns

- Don't use grease or ointments on severe burns.

- Cool partial-thickness or full-thickness burns with water only, not ice.

- Blisters are a natural cooling system. Leave them in place.

- Touch a burn only with sterile or clean dressings. Do not use absorbent cotton or pull clothes over any burned area.

- If the burn involves large areas of the head, face, hands, feet, or groin, seek medical attention.

Head and Spine Injuries

Head and Spine Injuries

An elderly woman is standing on a stepladder trying to reach the top shelf of a kitchen cupboard. She loses her balance and falls backwards, hitting her head on the counter as she falls.

Head and spine injuries can be fatal. People who survive can have physical difficulties and problems with how their brain works. This includes paralysis, speech and memory problems, and behavioural disorders. Head and spine injuries may lead to permanent disability.

 Causes

- Motor vehicle collisions
- Falls
- Recreation and sports injuries
- Violent acts, such as assault

You should suspect that there are head and/or spine injuries in the following situations:

- A fall from any height greater than the height of the person
- Any diving injury
- A person found unconscious for unknown reasons
- Any injury that involves a strong blow to the lower jaw, head, or trunk
- Any injury that causes a wound in the head or trunk
- A motor vehicle collision or rollover or ejection from a vehicle
- Any injury in which the person's helmet is damaged
- A lightning strike
- Electrocution

As a First Aider, you may not be able to determine how much damage has taken place without advanced medical assessment and diagnosis, so always treat the injury as if it were serious.

Prevention

- Always buckle up. Wear safety belts and shoulder restraints when you're in a vehicle.

- Babies and children should always ride in approved safety seats. Make sure the seat is designed for the child's age and weight and make sure it is properly installed.

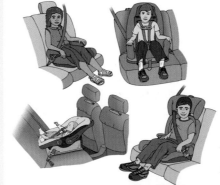

- For any activities for which you need protection, wear a properly fitting helmet approved by the Canadian Standards Association (CSA), proper eyewear, and other protective equipment. Helmets should fit comfortably and securely. All bicycle riders— adults, teens, and children— should wear a helmet.

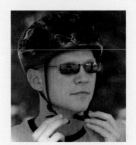

- Take safety precautions in all contact sports by wearing proper protection, such as mouthpieces, helmets, and eyewear.

- Never join in a new sport without knowing the rules and risks involved.

- Prevent falls around the home and workplace with non-slip floors, non-slip treads on stairs, handrails on staircases, rugs secured with double-sided adhesive tape, and handrails by the bathtub and toilet when necessary.

- Make sure that there is good lighting in stairways and hallways.

- If there are small children in your home, put gates at the top and bottom of the stairways.

- Make sure your workplace is clean and tidy. Keep floors and aisles uncluttered and make sure there is nothing blocking stairways, work sites, or exits.

- Drink responsibly. Alcohol is often a factor in serious motor vehicle collisions and water injuries. Alcohol slows down your reflexes and gives you a false feeling of confidence.

- Prescription drugs and common drugstore medications can also make driving or operating machinery dangerous, so follow the directions on the package carefully.

- Check equipment, such as warehouse forklifts, ladders, and scaffolding, regularly for worn or loose parts.
- Use ladders carefully and correctly.
- Always be very careful around water:
  - ▶ Before you dive, make sure the water is deep enough. Pools at homes, motels, or hotels may not be safe for diving.
  - ▶ Enter unknown water feet first.
  - ▶ Enter above-ground pools feet first.
  - ▶ Always swim with a buddy.
  - ▶ Before diving, check for objects below the surface, such as logs or pilings.
  - ▶ When you're bodysurfing, keep your arms in front of you to protect your head and neck.

▶ **What to Look For**

These signs and symptoms alone do not always mean a serious head and/or spine injury. However, you should always call EMS/9-1-1 when you suspect that there may be a serious head and/or spine injury.

- Changes in level of consciousness and behaviour
- Shock
- Drowsiness
- Severe pain or pressure in the head, neck, or back
- Blood or clear fluid coming from the ears or nose
- Heavy bleeding from the head, neck, or back
- Unusual bumps on the head, neck, or back
- Seizures
- Difficulty breathing or seeing properly
- Nausea or vomiting
- Unequal pupil size
- A headache that won't go away
- Weakness or an inability to use a leg or arm
- Numbness, tingling, or loss of feeling in any body part
- Unusually positioned neck or back
- Dizziness, disorientation, and/or loss of balance
- Bruising of the head, especially around the eyes and behind the ears
- Loss of bladder or bowel control

Bleeding inside the skull can happen slowly, so the symptoms may take time to appear.

 What to Do

Whenever you suspect that there might be a head and/or spine injury:

Check:

- Check the scene to ensure it is safe.
- If it is safe to do so, approach the person. Tell the person not to move. Make sure that your movements won't make the person's head or neck move. Then check the person and the person's ABCs.

Call:

- Have someone call EMS/9-1-1 and get an AED. If you are alone, call EMS/9-1-1 yourself, get an AED, and then return to care for the person.

Care:

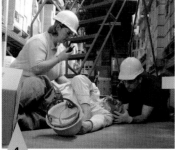

NOTE:
Remember your gloves and other barrier devices.

NOTE:
You can stabilize the spine and head when the person is lying down, sitting, or standing by holding his or her head with both of your hands.

1 Once you reach the person, make sure the head and spine move as little as possible by placing your hands on both sides of the person's head. Gently support the person's head in the position in which you found it until EMS personnel arrive.

2 If the person is wearing a helmet, leave it on unless it makes it difficult for you to ensure the ABCs are present.

3 If the ABCs are present, perform a secondary survey as best as you can without letting go of the person's head. If there is another First Aider or bystander, have him or her help you.

4 Provide continual care until EMS personnel arrive.

NOTE:
You don't always have to roll the person onto his or her back to check for breathing. If you hear a cry of pain, see chest movement, or hear the sound of breathing, it means the person is breathing.

NOTE:
If the person vomits, carefully roll him or her onto one side to keep the airway clear.

Leave the person in the position he or she was found unless the person is in immediate danger or has life-threatening conditions that need immediate attention.

Any injury that is serious enough to fracture or dislocate the jaw, nose, or other facial bones can cause other head and/or spine injuries.

A person who has no signs or symptoms may still have a head and/or spine injury. If the cause of the injury means that a head and/or spine injury is likely, treat the person as if he or she has one.

Unless you have the proper equipment and training to move a person with a suspected head and/or spine injury, wait for EMS personnel to arrive.

▶ Moving a Person With a Head and/or Spine Injury

A log roll (Figure 9.1) is the safest way to move a person with a head and/or spine injury. You should do this if:

- You need to clear the person's airway.

- You suspect a life-threatening injury on the back.

- You need to move the person onto something solid to remove them from a dangerous situation.

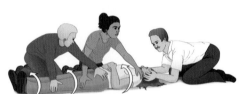

Figure 9.1 A log roll.

CONCUSSION

A **concussion** happens when a blow to the head or the body (e.g., whiplash) causes the brain to shake inside the skull. This can result in bleeding and/or swelling in or around the brain.

Concussions can be mild, serious, or somewhere in between.

▶ Causes

- A single, forceful movement of the head
- Several repeated, forceful movements of the head
- A violent blow to the lower jaw
- Shaking (in the case of a baby)
- An explosion
- A blunt force to the head
- A motor vehicle collision
- A forceful blow to the body

▶ What to Look For

- In most cases, if someone loses consciousness, it is for only a short period of time, although sometimes it lasts several minutes. It is a temporary condition.
- The person may say that he or she "blacked out" or "saw stars."
- Sometimes the person is confused or has memory loss.

> **NOTE:**
> The majority of concussions do not result in any altered level or loss of consciousness.

 ## What to Do

Follow the same Check, Call, Care steps as for head and spine injuries.

Shaken Baby Syndrome

When a baby won't stop crying, some people get so angry and frustrated that they shake the baby. This can cause fractures of the baby's skull, ribs, arms or legs; heavy bleeding; bruising; and brain swelling, which stops oxygen from getting to the brain. Seek medical attention immediately.

Shaken Baby Syndrome (SBS) can occur in babies and children between the ages of birth and five years. The majority of cases happen in babies less than six months old.

Often there is no intent to harm the child, but SBS is the most common cause of infant mortality. It is the most frequent cause of long-term disability in babies and young children.

Never shake a baby or a child, no matter what. Place the baby on his or her back in a safe place and let the baby cry while you take a few deep breaths and then try again to soothe the baby.

Contact your local help or crisis line if you need help to deal with anger or frustration.

SCALP INJURY

 ### What to Do

Check:

- Check the scene to ensure it is safe.
- If it is safe to do so, check the person and the person's ABCs.

Call:

- Call EMS/9-1-1 and get an AED if you are not sure how serious a scalp injury it is or if you feel a dip, a soft area, or pieces of bone.

Care:

- Ensure the person's ABCs are present.

- Perform a secondary survey and treat any non-life-threatening conditions. Pay particular attention to the area of injury because hair may be hiding part of the wound.

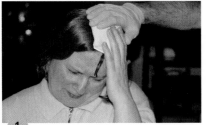

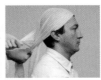

2 Secure the dressings with a bandage.

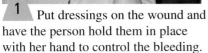

1 Put dressings on the wound and have the person hold them in place with her hand to control the bleeding.

If you feel a dip, a soft area, or pieces of bone:

1. Treat the injury as a head injury.

2. Put direct pressure on the wound only if the bleeding is severe.

3. Try to control the bleeding with pressure on the area around the wound.

4. Provide continual care until EMS personnel arrive.

NOTES:

Bone, Muscle, and Joint Injuries

Bone, Muscle, and Joint Injuries

A roofer is carrying a box of tools across the building site. He trips on a pile of lumber and falls forward, spraining his ankle and breaking a wrist.

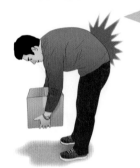

Strain—the stretching or tearing of muscles or **tendons**.

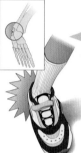

Sprain—the stretching or tearing of **ligaments** at a joint.

Dislocation—an injury that moves a bone out of its normal position at a joint.

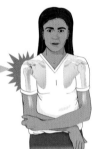

Fracture—a break, chip, or crack in a bone. In an open fracture, the bone breaks through the skin; in a closed fracture, the skin isn't broken.

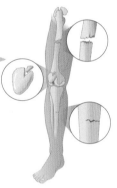

▶ Causes

Bone, muscle, and joint injuries can occur in many ways. The causes include:

- Falls
- Awkward or sudden movements
- Motor vehicle collisions
- A direct blow to the body
- Repetitive forces, such as running (stress fractures)
- Many contact and non-contact sports

▶ Prevention

- Always wear seat belts and shoulder restraints when you're in a vehicle.
- Small children must be in approved and properly installed child restraint systems (e.g., car seats, booster seats).
- During activities, wear the appropriate safety equipment correctly (e.g., helmets, goggles, and pads).
- When you are bicycling, always wear an approved bicycle helmet.
- Put non-slip adhesive strips or a mat in the bath.
- Wear proper protection correctly when you're playing contact sports.
- Know the risks and rules of new sports and jobs.
- Check the water depth before diving.
- Enter above-ground pools feet first.
- Stretch before exercising.
- Know your limits. When you are too tired or frustrated, take a break.

Falls are the leading cause of injuries among the elderly. Reduce the risk with safety measures such as:

- Good lighting
- Sturdy railings on staircases
- Non-slip floors and rugs

▶ What to Look For

- Pain
- Deformity
- Swelling
- Bruising
- Limited use of, or inability to move, the injured body part due to pain
- A broken bone or bone fragments sticking out of the skin or wound
- A sensation or sound of bones grating
- Possible muscle cramps
- The sound of a snap or a pop when the injury happened
- Shock

> **NOTE:**
>
> Bone, muscle, and joint injuries are almost always painful. Without first aid, they can lead to serious injuries and even permanent disabilities. In some cases, they can be life-threatening.

A muscle cramp is not actually an injury. It is a painful condition that can be caused by heavy exercise or by staying in the same position for too long. You can usually stop the pain by:

- Resting

- Stretching and massaging the area with the cramp

- Changing the position of the area with the cramp

 ## What to Do

Check:

- Check the scene to ensure it is safe.

- If it is safe to do so, check the person and the person's ABCs.

NOTE:

If you expect the ambulance will arrive in a few minutes, keep the person still and do not splint the injury. If the ambulance is going to take longer to arrive, immobilize the injury in the position found if it does not cause further damage or pain.

Call:

- Call EMS/9-1-1 and get an AED when:

  ▶ There is a problem with the ABCs.

  ▶ The injury involves the head and/or spine.

  ▶ The injury makes walking difficult.

  ▶ You suspect that there may be more than one injury.

  ▶ There are injuries to the thigh bone or **pelvis**.

  ▶ The person has an altered level of consciousness.

Care:

- Ensure the person's ABCs are present.

- Perform a secondary survey and treat any non-life-threatening conditions:

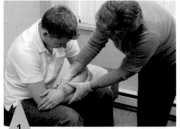

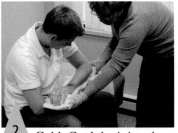

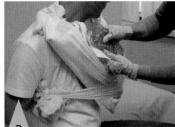

1 Treat the injury using the RICE method:

Rest: Have the person stop what he was doing.

Immobilize: Immobilize the injured area in the position in which it was found.

2 **C**old: Cool the injured area for 20 minutes of every hour for the first 24 to 48 hours. If you use ice, put some sort of thin cloth or pad between it and the bare skin to avoid freezing the skin.

3 **E**levate: Keep the injured area above the level of the heart if possible. However, do not raise the injured area if moving it will cause pain.

4 Provide continual care.

R - **Rest**

I - **Immobilize**

C - **Cold**

E - **Elevate**

> **NOTE:**
>
> **Remember your gloves and other barrier devices.**

Splinting Guidelines

There are four types of **splints**:

- **Soft splints** include folded blankets, towels, pillows, and bandages.

- **Rigid splints** immobilize an injured body part by securing it to something rigid, such as a board, a rolled newspaper, a tree branch, etc.

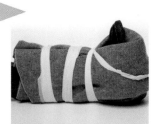

- **Anatomical splints** use another body part for support. For example, you could immobilize an injured leg by securing it to the uninjured leg.

- **Slings** are looped around the neck to support an arm, hand, or wrist.

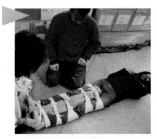

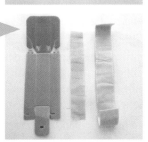

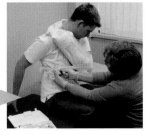

No matter what type of splint you use, follow these steps:

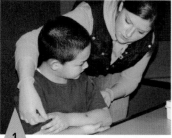

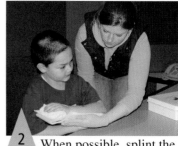

1 Check for skin temperature and colour below the injured area before and after splinting. The area should be warm, indicating good circulation. If the area is cold before splinting, seek medical attention quickly. If the area was warm before splinting and cold afterwards, the splint may be too tight. Loosen it gently.

2 When possible, splint the injured part in the position in which it was found.

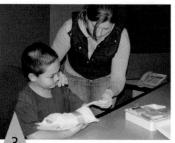

4 Always pad a rigid or anatomical splint to make the person more comfortable.

3 For bone and joint injuries, immobilize above and below the site of the injury.

Applying a regular sling and binder:

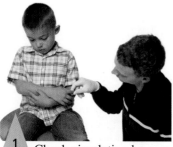

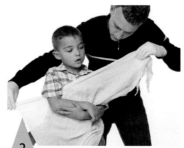

1 Check circulation by comparing the warmth and colour of the fingers with the other hand.

- Remove any rings the person is wearing.

- Ask the person if he has any numbness or tingling in the fingers.

2 From the most comfortable position, have the person support the injured arm, holding it across the body with the fingers pointed at the opposite shoulder.

- Position the open triangular bandage under the injured arm, against the body. The point of the triangular bandage should extend past the elbow. The opposite, or bottom, end should be straight up and down on the body with the upper end over the shoulder.

- Take the bottom end of the bandage and place it over the opposite shoulder.

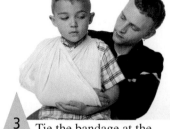 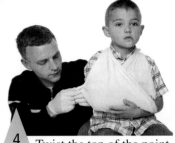 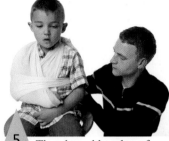

3 Tie the bandage at the back of the neck, making sure that the knot does not create any discomfort.

4 Twist the top of the point of the bandage.

5 Tie a broad bandage from the elbow on the injured side across the body.

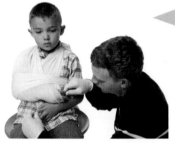

6 Recheck circulation by checking the colour and warmth of the fingers.

- Ask the person if he has any numbness or tingling in the fingers.
- Slings should fit tight enough to restrict movement, but not so tight that blood flow is affected.

Applying a tube sling for a collarbone fracture:

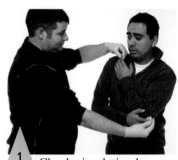 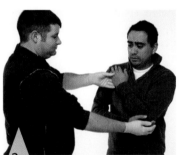 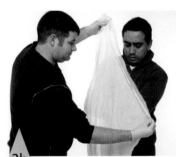

1 Check circulation by comparing the warmth and colour of the fingers with the other hand.

- Remove any rings the person is wearing.
- Ask the person if he has any numbness or tingling in the fingers.

2a Put the forearm of the injured side across the chest, with fingers pointing at the opposite arm.

2b Position the open triangular bandage over the forearm and hand.

- The point of the triangular bandage should extend past the elbow and shoulder.

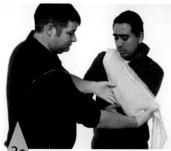

2c Support the forearm and carefully tuck the bandage under all the way from the hand to the elbow.

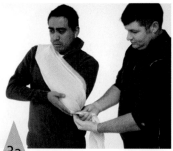

3a Carry the end of the bandage near the elbow around the back.
- Twist the top of the point of the bandage near the elbow to secure the elbow from coming out of the sling.

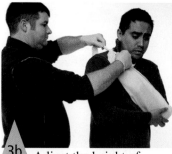

3b Adjust the height of the sling to make sure it is supporting the arm.
- Tie the ends together in the hollow of the neck on the uninjured side.

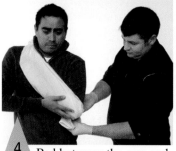

4 Pad between the arm and the body, in the natural hollow, with soft, firm material.

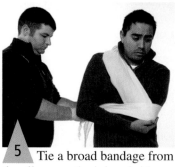

5 Tie a broad bandage from the elbow on the injured side across the body.

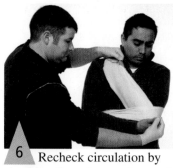

6 Recheck circulation by checking the colour and warmth of the fingers.
- Ask the person if he has any numbness or tingling in the fingers.
- Slings should fit tight enough to restrict movement, but not so tight that blood flow is affected.

> If fingers are bluish or cold or if the person feels numbness and tingling, loosen the bandages. If loosening the bandages does not improve circulation, call EMS/9-1-1 and get an AED immediately.

OSTEOPOROSIS

Osteoporosis is a leading cause of bone and joint injuries in older people. It happens when the amount of calcium in your bones decreases, making the bones frail. It is not usually discovered until after age 65, but it can begin at a very early age. Osteoporosis affects one in four women, but it is less common in men.

▶ **Prevention**

- Build strong bones at an early age.
- Make sure you get enough calcium.
- Make sure you get enough vitamin D (your body needs vitamin D so that it can absorb calcium).
- Exercise regularly.

Talk to your doctor about testing and treatment for osteoporosis.

▶ **What to Look For**

- Fractures occur with little or no external force.
- Fractures of the hips, **vertebrae**, and wrists are particularly common.

NOTE:

Often osteoporosis is not diagnosed until after a fracture occurs.

NOTES:

Sudden Medical Emergencies

Sudden Medical Emergencies

You are standing in line at the bank behind a 23-year-old woman who is eight months pregnant. Suddenly, she collapses onto the floor.

FAINTING

Fainting is a brief period of unconsciousness that happens when there isn't enough blood flowing to the brain.

 Causes

- Pregnancy
- Standing in one position for too long without moving
- Pain
- Traumatic information, such as news of someone's death
- Heat
- Dehydration
- Not eating enough

 Prevention

- Watch for the warning signs of fainting, such as dizziness or nausea, and sit or lie down.
- Keep hydrated and nourished.
- Wear loose clothing around the neck.
- When standing up from sitting or laying down, do so slowly.

 What to Do

Check:

- Check the scene to ensure it is safe.
- If it is safe to do so, check the person and the person's ABCs.

Call:

- Call EMS/9-1-1 and get an AED.

Care:

1. Ensure the person's ABCs are present.

2. Perform a secondary survey and treat any non-life-threatening conditions:

   - Place the person in the recovery position so that blood can start flowing to the brain again and the airway stays open.

3. If the person is pregnant, has a history of heart disease, or has another serious illness, seek medical attention.

DIABETIC EMERGENCIES

A **diabetic emergency** happens when the body cannot control the level of sugar in the blood. The blood sugar level may become too high (**hyperglycemia**) or too low (**hypoglycemia**). Hyperglycemia develops slowly, so it is less likely to be a first aid emergency.

> **NOTE:**
> Not all people with a blood sugar emergency have diabetes.

Causes

- An imbalance between two or more of the following:

  - ▶ Exercise

  - ▶ Food intake

  - ▶ **Insulin** production

Prevention

- Take your medications as prescribed.

- Check your blood sugar often, especially if you are sick or not following your normal routine.

- Keep some quick-sugar foods with you at all times.

What to Look For

- Changes in the level of consciousness

- Changes in behaviour, such as confusion or aggression

- Rapid breathing

- Cool, sweaty skin

- Skin that is paler than normal

- Appearance of intoxication

- Feeling and looking ill

NOTE:

Some people with diabetes wear a MedicAlert® medical identification product (see Chapter 4).

You don't need to know the difference between the two types of diabetic emergencies (hyperglycemia and hypoglycemia) because first aid is the same for both.

 ## What to Do

Check:

• Check the scene to ensure it is safe.

• If it is safe to do so, check the person and the person's ABCs.

Call:

• Call EMS/9-1-1 and get an AED.

Care:

1. Ensure the person's ABCs are present.

2. Perform a secondary survey and treat any non-life-threatening conditions:

   • If the person is conscious (and the person knows it is a diabetic emergency):

      ▶ Offer the person a sugary drink such as orange or apple juice.

      ▶ If the person's condition improves, recommend he or she eat a complete meal.

   • If the person is unconscious:

      ▶ Perform a secondary survey and place the person in the recovery position.

      ▶ Provide continual care until EMS personnel arrive.

SEIZURES

A seizure is an episode of abnormal electrical signals in the brain that result in disturbed brain function, shaking or contraction of limbs, and altered consciousness.

 Causes

- Head injuries
- Fever
- Certain medical conditions
- **Poisons** (including drugs)
- Drug or alcohol withdrawal
- Heat stroke
- Certain video games or other audiovisual stimulation that involves flashes
- Infection

 Prevention

- Follow the guidelines throughout this manual for preventing injuries at work, home, or play.
- If you have seizures, take your prescribed medication regularly.
- If a child has a fever, make sure it doesn't get too high. If a child's fever is higher than a fever caused by a normal cold or flu, seek medical attention.
- Limit the amount of time spent playing video games.

BABY OR CHILD WITH A FEVER OVER 39°C (102°F)

 What to Do

Young children or babies with a high fever can have seizures. In most cases these are not life-threatening and they do not last long. To prevent seizures:

1. Give the child medication recommended by the child's doctor to reduce the fever.
2. Give the child a sponge bath with water that is room temperature (not icy cold).
3. Provide continual care.

Since these steps only temporarily lower the temperature, seek medical attention.

What to Look For

- A sense of urgency to get to safety
- Hallucinations such as seeing, hearing, tasting, or smelling something that doesn't actually exist
- Appearance of daydreaming
- Uncontrollable muscle movement
- Eyes rolling upward, back into the head
- Drool or foam in the mouth

 What to Do

Check:

- Check the scene to ensure it is safe.
- If it is safe to do so, check the person and the person's ABCs.

Call:

Call EMS/9-1-1 and get an AED if:

- The seizure lasts more than a few minutes.
- The person has several seizures in a row.
- The person appears to be injured.
- You are not sure what caused the seizure.
- The person is pregnant.
- The person has diabetes.
- The person is a baby or a child.
- The seizure takes place in water.
- The person doesn't wake up after the seizure.

Care:

During the seizure:

 1 Never put anything in the person's mouth.

 2 Allow the person to move without restraint.

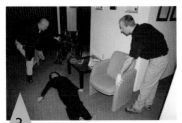 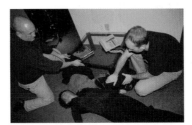

3 Protect the person from injury by:
  • Moving furniture
  • Protecting the person's head with blankets
  • Keeping other dangers away from the person

After the seizure:

1. Ensure the person's ABCs are present.
2. Perform a secondary survey and treat any non-life-threatening conditions:
   • Make sure there aren't any fluids in the person's mouth.
   • Place the person in the recovery position.
   • Keep the person comfortable and warm.
3. Provide continual care.

CHILDBIRTH

NOTE:

Women who have had children previously often have a shorter labour.

 What to Look For

- **Contractions** are two minutes apart or less.
- The woman says that the baby is coming.
- The baby's head is showing.

 What to Do

Check:

- Check the scene to ensure it is safe.
- If it is safe to do so, check the woman and her ABCs.

Call:

- Have someone call EMS/9-1-1 and get an AED. If you are alone, call EMS/9-1-1 yourself, get an AED, and then return to care for the woman.

Care:

1. Ensure the woman's ABCs are present.

2. Help the woman to be as comfortable and calm as possible.

3. Wash your hands and wear gloves.

4. Put clean towels, a blanket, or any available material under her buttocks.

5. As the baby's head comes out, support it with one hand. Do not push or pull the baby. Once the shoulders come out, be prepared for the rest of the baby to come out very quickly. Newborns are slippery, so hold the baby firmly but do not squeeze.

6. Place the baby face down and ensure that the baby's ABCs are present.

7. Keep the baby warm by wrapping the baby in a clean cloth.

NOTE:

Give the woman as much privacy as possible.

NOTE:

Throughout the process continue to give the woman encouragement and reassurance.

8. Let the placenta and cord drop onto a clean towel and keep this near the baby. Do not cut the cord.

9. If the mother keeps bleeding, you may need to apply gentle pressure to any bleeding tears.

10. Treat the mother and baby for shock.

11. Provide continual care for both mother and baby until EMS personnel arrive.

> **NOTE:**
>
> Remember your gloves and other barrier devices.

Be prepared to start CPR (see Chapter 7) or **rescue breathing** (for healthcare providers: see Chapter 14) if the baby doesn't start breathing.

MISCARRIAGE

Miscarriage is the spontaneous termination of a pregnancy in the first 20 weeks after conception. The risk of miscarriage drops as the pregnancy progresses.

▶ Causes

There are a number of causes of miscarriage. Some of these include:

- Hormonal or genetic reasons
- Abnormalities in the womb
- Infection
- Certain illnesses
- Age
- Trauma

Prevention

- Talk to your doctor about what you can do to reduce the risks of a preventable miscarriage.

What to Look For

- Anxiety

- Vaginal bleeding

- Cramp-like pain that is similar to **labour** or menstruation

 What to Do

Check:

- Check the scene to ensure it is safe.

- If it is safe to do so, check the woman and her ABCs.

Call:

- Have someone call EMS/9-1-1 and get an AED. If you are alone, call EMS/9-1-1 yourself, get an AED, and then return to care for the woman.

Care:

1. Ensure the woman's ABCs are present.

2. Attempt to calm and comfort the woman.

3. Perform a secondary survey and treat any non-life-threatening conditions.

4. Provide continual care until EMS personnel arrive.

Environmental Emergencies

Environmental Emergencies

A 55-year-old moose hunter has a few drinks to keep warm while he is out in the woods on an October afternoon. On his way back to his cabin, he slips and falls in a creek. It takes him more than two hours to get back. When he arrives he is shivering, his hands and feet are numb, and he has difficulty speaking.

Cold-Related Emergencies

FROST NIP AND FROSTBITE

Frost nip is a superficial injury caused by freezing of the skin (Figure 12.1). In a case of **frostbite**, the tissue underneath the skin freezes as well (Figure 12.2). Your extremities, such as your ears, fingers, and nose, are particularly prone to frostbite. Frostbite is often associated with hypothermia.

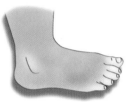

Figure 12.1 Frost nip.

 Causes

* Exposure to cold temperatures

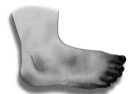

Figure 12.2 Frostbite.

 Prevention

* If you are in, on, or around a cold environment, prepare properly, wear layers of clothing, and warm yourself if you feel cold.

* Wear a hat and layers of clothing made of tightly woven fibres, such as wool, or synthetics, such as fleece, which trap warm air against your body. AVOID COTTON!

* Cover up vulnerable areas such as your fingers, toes, cheeks, ears, and nose (but don't cover them too tightly).

* Drink plenty of warm fluids to help your body stay warm. If warm drinks are not available, drink plenty of plain water.

- Avoid caffeine and alcohol because they can cause dehydration, which stops your body from controlling its temperature properly.

- Take frequent breaks from the cold to let your body warm up. This will help you cope better with short periods of extreme cold.

▶ What to Look For

Frost Nip

- Pain or stinging in the area, followed by numbness

- Skin that looks paler than the area around it

Frostbite

- Waxy skin that is colder than the area around it

- Skin that is hard and solid to the touch

- After thawing, there may be a burning sensation, redness, pain, and tenderness, and blisters may form

 ## What to Do

Check:

- Check the scene to ensure it is safe.

- If it is safe to do so, check the person and the person's ABCs.

Call:

- Call EMS/9-1-1 and get an AED if the frost nip or frostbite is combined with severe **hypothermia**. See "Hypothermia" in this chapter.

Care:

1. Remove the person from the cold environment.

2. Ensure the person's ABCs are present.

3. Perform a secondary survey and treat any non-life-threatening conditions:

   - Warm the affected area gradually using warm water or body heat.

   - Don't break any blisters! Protect them with loose, dry dressings. Place gauze between the fingers or toes if they are affected.

4. If you suspect that the person may have frostbite, seek medical attention.

Don't rub the frozen area or put snow on it. Warm the area only if you are sure it will not freeze again.

SNOW BLINDNESS

 ## Causes

Looking at snow for too long on a bright day can damage your eyes, causing snow blindness. That's because the snow reflects the sun's ultraviolet rays.

 ### Prevention

- Wear sunglasses when you are outdoors in the snow in the daytime. Choose a pair that:
  - ▶ Prevents light from shining in from underneath or above or from the sides.
  - ▶ Blocks 100 percent of the UV rays

 ## What to Look For

- Redness
- Swelling of the tissue around the eyes
- Pain, itchiness, or a burning sensation in the eyes that may become intense

 ## What to Do

Check:

- Check the scene to ensure it is safe.
- If it is safe to do so, check the person and the person's ABCs.

Call:

- Call EMS/9-1-1 only if you are unable to get the person to medical attention.

Care:

1. Ensure the person's ABCs are present.
2. Perform a secondary survey and treat any non-life-threatening conditions:
   - Place the person in a darker environment.
   - Use cool, damp cloths to reduce pain and burning.
3. Seek medical attention.

The symptoms of snow blindness may not appear for several hours following exposure to bright, snowy conditions.

HYPOTHERMIA

Hypothermia is a life-threatening condition that develops when a person's body temperature drops too low.

 ## Causes

- Exposure to cold temperatures for too long

People at Risk of Hypothermia

- People who work or exercise outdoors
- Elderly people
- Young children
- People who do not consume enough calories
- People who are dehydrated
- People with health problems
- People who have had a **heat-related emergency** or **cold-related emergency** in the past
- People who have heart disease or other conditions that cause poor circulation
- People who take medications to eliminate water from the body

 ## Prevention

- Check the weather forecast before you plan outdoor activities.
- If you are in, on, or around a cold environment, prepare properly, wear layers of clothing, and warm yourself if you feel cold.
- Wear a hat and layers of clothing made of tightly woven fibres, such as wool, or synthetics, such as fleece, which trap warm air against your body. Wool insulates you even when it is wet. AVOID COTTON!
- Cover up vulnerable areas such as your fingers, toes, cheeks, ears, and nose (but don't cover them too tightly).
- Cover up your head and trunk because you lose most of your heat from these areas.

- Shivering is your body's first response to cold. Blue lips and vigorous shivering are warning signs of hypothermia.

- As soon as you start shivering, get out of the cold and let your body warm up. This will help you cope better with short periods of extreme cold.

- Drink plenty of warm fluids to help your body stay warm. If warm drinks are not available, drink plenty of plain water.

- Avoid caffeine and alcohol because they cause dehydration, which stops your body from controlling its temperature properly. Carry a high-energy food that has a lot of sugar.

- Carry a lighter or matches in a waterproof container. You may need to build a fire to warm up.

- When you are boating or on the water, wear a properly sized personal flotation device (PFD) or lifejacket

- Be extremely careful around water. Hypothermia can occur in any body of water, warm or cold.

- If your clothes get wet when you are in the cold, change into dry clothing immediately.

▶ Things to Remember

- Hypothermia can be mild, moderate, or severe (Table 12.1).

- Hypothermia can get worse very quickly if the person is wet and the environment is cold.

- Hypothermia can slowly get worse if the person is dry but the environment is cold.

- Hypothermia can occur at any time of the year.

Table 12.1 Hypothermia

Level of Severity	What to Look For	NOTE:
Mild	Shivering and complaining of the cold Numbness Body temperature slightly below normal	Normal body temperature is 37°C (98.6°F).
Moderate	Shivering and sometimes complaining of the cold Numbness Lack of coordination and/or speech Confused or unusual behaviour Impaired judgment	
Severe	Person has stopped shivering Person has stopped complaining of the cold Numbness Lack of coordination and/or speech Confused or unusual behaviour Impaired judgment Body temperature below 30°C (86°F) Breathing that has slowed down or stopped Possible unconsciousness Body that feels stiff	

37
36 Mild
35
34 Moderate
33
32
31
30 Severe
29
28
27
°C

 What to Do

Check:

- Check the scene to ensure it is safe.
- If it is safe to do so, check the person and the person's ABCs.

Call:

- Call EMS/9-1-1 and get an AED for severe hypothermia.

Care:

1. Ensure the person's ABCs are present.

2. Treat the person very gently and monitor breathing carefully.

3. Get the person away from the cold and into some kind of shelter, if possible.

4. Remove any wet clothing and dry the person.

5. Warm the person by wrapping him or her in blankets or putting on dry clothing. Cover the head and neck. Warm the person slowly. Warming too quickly can cause heart problems.

6. If hot water bottles, heating pads, or other heat sources are available, put them in each armpit, the groin, and the back of the neck. If you use a heating pad, make sure the person is dry. Keep a blanket, towel, or clothing between the heat source and the skin to avoid burns. Active re-warming should be used only when the person is far from a medical facility.

7. If the person is alert, give him or her warm liquids to drink (no alcohol or caffeine).

8. Perform a secondary survey and treat any non-life-threatening conditions.

9. Provide continual care until EMS personnel arrive.

NOTE:

For Healthcare Providers: If the person is unconscious, take up to 45 seconds to check for signs of circulation. Perform rescue breathing if necessary.

FREEZING OF SKIN TO METAL OBJECTS

The tongue, lips, and other moist parts of skin can freeze to cold metal objects.

 ### Causes

- Freezing of moist skin to a cold metal object

 ### What to Do

Check:

- Check the scene to ensure it is safe.

- If it is safe to do so, check the person and the person's ABCs.

Call:

- Call EMS/9-1-1 and get an AED if you cannot safely remove the body part from the object.

Care:

1. Ensure the person's ABCs are present.

2. Pour warm water on the surface of the object and/or the skin that is stuck to the object. Do not use hot water!

3. Gradually and gently help release the person from the metal object.

4. Perform a secondary survey and treat any non-life-threatening conditions:

    • Treat any torn skin as an open wound.

5. Provide continual care.

Heat-Related Emergencies

 ## Causes

Causes/risk factors that increase the likelihood of **heat exhaustion**, **heat stroke**, and other heat-related illnesses (Table 12.2) can be broken into four areas[2]:

1. Environmental:

    • Heat waves, especially if there hasn't been one in recent years

    • High humidity (above 75 percent), which decreases people's ability to sweat

2. Physical:

    • Age: babies, children, and the elderly are less able to sweat and adjust to changes in temperature

    • Chronic illness

    • Heart disease

    • Certain skin, hormone, or nervous system diseases

    • Burns

3. Behavioural:

    • Spending too much time in the heat or sun

    • Not drinking enough fluids (Figure 12.3) to replace the water lost by sweating (dehydration)

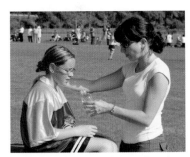

Figure 12.3 Drink plenty of cool fluids.

[2]Adapted from Robert S. Helman, MD. *Heatstroke*. Available at www.emedicine.com (accessed December 2010).

- Working or exercising too much in hot weather
- Drinking too much alcohol in hot weather
- Taking drugs such as cocaine, amphetamines, or other stimulants

4. Others:
   - Salt depletion or water depletion
   - Obesity
   - Fatigue
   - Poor physical fitness

▶ **Prevention**

- Drink plenty of cool fluids—this is the most important action you can take to prevent heat-related emergencies.
- Avoid being outdoors during the hottest part of the day.
- Slow down your activities as it gets hotter and don't work or exercise for too long at a time.
- Take frequent breaks in a cool or shaded area to let your body cool off. This will help you cope better with short periods of extreme heat.
- Dress for the heat and for your activity level.
- Wear a hat when you're in the sun. Wear light-coloured cotton clothing to absorb sweat and let air circulate and heat escape.
- Avoid caffeine and alcohol because they can cause dehydration, which stops your body from controlling its temperature properly.

NOTE:

People at risk of heat-related emergencies are the same as those who are at risk of cold-related emergencies.

Table 12.2 Heat-Related Emergencies

Type of Injury	What to Look For	What to Do
Heat cramps	Mild muscle contractions that can become severe, usually in the legs and abdomen but can be in other body parts Normal body temperature (37°C or 98.6°F) in most cases Moist skin	**Check:** • Check the scene to ensure it is safe. • If it is safe to do so, check the person and the person's ABCs. **Call:** • Call for someone to get cool water. **Care:** 1. Ensure the person's ABCs are present. 2. Have the person rest in a cool place. 3. Give the person fluids to drink, preferably juices or sports drinks. 4. Perform a secondary survey and treat any non-life-threatening conditions: • Gently stretch and massage the cramped muscles. 5. Provide continual care.

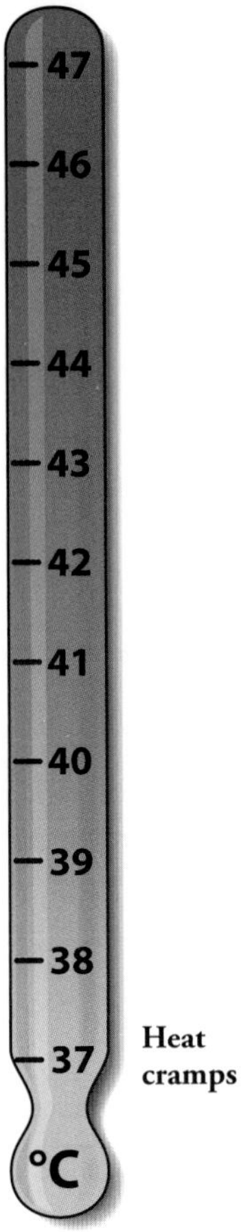

47
46
45
44
43
42
41
40
39
38
37

Heat cramps

°C

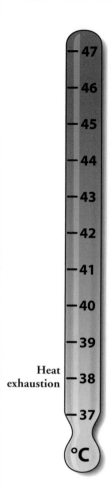

Heat
exhaustion

°C

Type of Injury	What to Look For	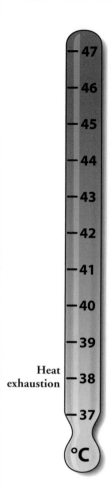 What to Do
Heat exhaustion	Normal or slightly raised body temperature (higher than 37°C or 98.6°F) Moist skin Skin that is redder or paler than normal Nausea Dizziness and weakness Exhaustion	**Check:** • Check the scene to ensure it is safe. • If it is safe to do so, check the person and the person's ABCs. **Call:** • Call EMS/9-1-1 and get an AED if the person is vomiting or is losing consciousness. **Care:** 1. Ensure the person's ABCs are present. 2. Have the person rest in a cool place. 3. Have the person loosen any tight clothing and if you are fanning the person remove any clothing that is soaked with sweat. 4. Put cool water on the skin and fan the person to increase evaporation. Avoid using any other substances on the skin. 5. If the person is conscious, have him or her take small sips of cool water. 6. Perform a secondary survey and treat any non-life-threatening conditions. 7. Don't let the person do any more activities in the heat that day. 8. If the condition gets worse, follow the treatment for heat stroke.

Type of Injury	What to Look For	🧰 What to Do
Heat stroke	High body temperature, often as high as 41°C (106°F)	**Check:** • Check the scene to ensure it is safe. • If it is safe to do so, check the person and the person's ABCs.
	Red, hot, dry skin, especially in the elderly	**Call:** • Have someone call EMS/9-1-1 and get an AED. If you are alone, call EMS/9-1-1 yourself, get an AED, and then return to care for the person.
	Irritable, bizarre, or aggressive behaviour	
	Progressive loss of consciousness	**Care:** 1. Ensure the person's ABCs are present.
	Rapid, weak **pulse** becoming irregular	2. Have the person rest in a cool place.
	Rapid, shallow breathing	3. Cool the body any way you can. Immerse the body in cool water from the neck down. Or you can sponge the entire body with tepid or cool water, fan the person, or put covered ice packs in the groin, in each armpit, and on the back of the neck to cool large blood vessels.
	Seizures	
		4. If the person is conscious, have him or her take small sips of cool water.
		5. Perform a secondary survey and treat any non-life-threatening conditions.
		6. Provide continual care until EMS personnel arrive.

47
46
45
44
43
42
41 — Heat stroke
40
39
38
37
°C

Heat-related emergencies will get worse without treatment and can change from one level to another very quickly.

DROWNING

 ## Causes

- Being submerged in water, which does not allow oxygen to get into the lungs or body

 ### Prevention

- Check the water depth before you swim or dive.
- Be prepared before you go in or on water. Bring any safety equipment you need.
- Know what to do to stay safe in, on, and around the water.
- Supervise children in, on, or around all water.
- Take Canadian Red Cross swimming and water safety lessons.

CONSCIOUS, DROWNING PERSON

 ## What to Look for

- Struggling and panicking in the water

 ## What to Do

Check:

- Check the scene to ensure it is safe.

Call:

- Have someone call EMS/9-1-1 and get an AED. If you are alone, call EMS/9-1-1 yourself and get an AED.

NOTE:

For Healthcare Providers: If you have special training, you can start rescue breathing while the person is still in the water if it does not delay removing the person from the water.

Care:

1. Remove the person quickly and safely from the water but do not put yourself in danger. Try to use a reaching assist while you stay in a safe position (see "Assisting a Conscious, Drowning Person With a Reaching Assist" in Chapter 3).

2. Ensure the person's ABCs are present.

3. You may need to treat the person for hypothermia.

4. Perform a secondary survey and treat any non-life-threatening conditions.

5. Provide continual care until EMS personnel arrive.

Poisons

Poisons

You're waiting for a haircut at a busy salon when you hear someone scream in the back. A stylist is grabbing one of her eyes. An open bottle of bleaching product is lying on the counter next to her, and the bleach is splattered everywhere.

A poison is a substance that has a harmful effect within the body if it is inhaled, swallowed, absorbed, or injected. Poisons are immediately life-threatening if they affect breathing or circulation. When you treat someone who has been poisoned, you should take precautions to make sure that you do not come in contact with the poison yourself.

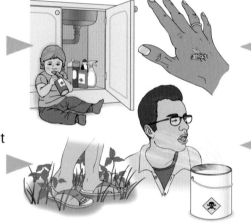

Swallowed (ingested) poisons come in contact with the mouth or lips.

Injected poisons enter the body through bites or stings or as drugs injected with a needle.

Absorbed poisons get into the body through the skin. Chemicals and plants can cause this type of poisoning.

Inhaled poisons are breathed into the body.

 Prevention

- Keep all medications, household products, poisonous plants, and other toxic substances well out of the reach of children. Use locked cupboards or special child-resistant latches.

- Treat all household or drugstore products as if they could be dangerous.

- Use child-resistant safety caps on medications and other potentially toxic products.

- Teach children to check with an adult before eating an unknown substance.

- Never call medicine "candy" to persuade a child to take it.

- Keep products in their original containers with their original labels.

- Use poison symbols to identify dangerous substances and teach children what the symbols mean.

- All medicine bottles and boxes should be carefully labelled. Read the label three times when you are taking or giving medication: 1) when you take the medication from the cupboard or refrigerator, 2) when you take the medication out of the package, 3) just before you administer the medication.

- Prescription medicine should be taken only by the person for whom it was prescribed.

- Carefully dispose of outdated medications by giving them to the pharmacist.

- When you're using chemicals that might be dangerous, work in a well-ventilated area and follow the instructions on the package carefully.

- Wear proper protective clothing any time you may come into contact with a poisonous substance.

- Keep the local Poison Control Centre number by your telephone.

- Run any gas engine only in an open space.

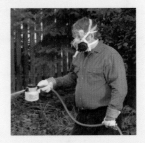

- Many cleaning products have toxic fumes. Read their labels and don't use them in confined areas.

- Mixing certain household cleaning products, such as bleach and household cleaner, can create toxic fumes.

- Use aerosol sprays only in open spaces.

- Learn about poisonous plants before you go hiking.

 Prevention in the Workplace

About one-quarter of all workers are exposed to chemical hazards in their workplace. According to WHMIS regulations, employers must:

- Clearly label hazardous materials, including all toxic substances.

- Tell employees about risks and precautions.

- Have a detailed MSDS available for every hazardous substance in the workplace.

- Give workers who may be exposed to hazardous materials the proper training in safety measures and emergency procedures.

Employees should:

- Check all warning labels, tags, and posters in the workplace and follow the instructions carefully.

- Read labels and MSDSs to find out the risks of each hazardous material, the safety measures to prevent poisoning, and the first aid for poisoning.
- Never use a product that is in an unidentified bottle.

Many everyday substances can be poisonous in large enough quantities.

SWALLOWED POISONS

 What to Look For

- An open container of poison nearby
- Burns around the mouth
- Increased production of saliva and/or saliva that is an abnormal colour
- Abdominal cramps and vomiting
- Seizures
- Dizziness and/or drowsiness
- Unconsciousness
- A burning sensation in the mouth, throat, or stomach
- Diarrhea

 What to Do

Check:
- Check the scene to ensure it is safe.
- If it is safe to do so, check the person and the person's ABCs.

Call:
- Call your local Poison Control Centre if the person is conscious and alert and the person's ABCs are present.
- Call EMS/9-1-1 and get an AED if the person has an altered level of consciousness or has difficulty breathing.

Care:
1. Ensure the person's ABCs are present.
2. Perform a secondary survey and treat any non-life-threatening conditions:

- Check the packaging of the poison, if possible, so that you know what it is.
- Induce vomiting only if told to do so by the EMS dispatcher or the Poison Control Centre.

3. Provide continual care.

4. If the person needs to go to the hospital, bring the container as well.

INHALED POISONS

 What to Look For

- Breathing difficulties
- Dizziness
- Seizures
- Unconsciousness
- A cloud in the air

- Irritated eyes, nose, or throat
- Vomiting
- Bluish colour around the mouth
- An unusual smell in the air

 What to Do

Check:

- Check the scene to ensure it is safe.
- If it is safe to do so, check the person and the person's ABCs.

Call:

- Call your local Poison Control Centre if the person is conscious and alert and the person's ABCs are present.
- Call EMS/9-1-1 and get an AED if the person has an altered level of consciousness or has difficulty breathing.

Care:

1. Ensure the person's ABCs are present.

2. Get the person into fresh air, but DO NOT enter into a hazardous atmosphere yourself to do so.

3. Perform a secondary survey and treat any non-life-threatening conditions.

4. Provide continual care.

> **NOTE:**
>
> If the person is not breathing, start CPR. Remember to use a barrier device so that you don't contaminate yourself with the poison.

Inhaled poisons can affect everyone in the area. Stay out of the area if you suspect that the poison may still be there.

ABSORBED POISONS

▶ **What to Look For**

- Rash
- Swelling
- Hives (raised, itchy areas of skin)
- Unconsciousness

- Burning, itching
- Blisters
- Burns

 What to Do

Check:

- Check the scene to ensure it is safe.
- If it is safe to do so, check the person and the person's ABCs.

Call:

- Call your local Poison Control Centre if the person is conscious and alert and the person's ABCs are present.
- Call EMS/9-1-1 and get an AED if the person has an altered level of consciousness or has difficulty breathing.

Care:

1 Ensure the person's ABCs are present.

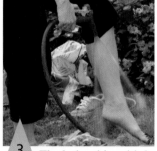

2 Remove the substance from the skin.

3 Flush the skin with large amounts of water for at least 15 minutes. To prevent any further injury, make sure the water flushes away from any unaffected areas of the body.

4 Perform a secondary survey and treat any non-life-threatening conditions.

5 Provide continual care.

INJECTED POISONS

 What to Look For

- Puncture wound
- Pain
- Redness and swelling at the entry point
- Problems breathing
- Prescription medications or illegal drugs nearby

 What to Do

Check:

- Check the scene to ensure it is safe.
- If it is safe to do so, check the person and the person's ABCs.

Call:

- Call your local Poison Control Centre if the person is conscious and alert and the person's ABCs are present.
- Call EMS/9-1-1 and get an AED if the person has an altered level of consciousness or has difficulty breathing.

Care:

1. Ensure the person's ABCs are present.
2. Keep the site of the puncture lower than the heart.
3. Have the person rest in a comfortable position.
4. Perform a secondary survey and treat any non-life-threatening conditions.
5. Provide continual care.

STINGS AND INSECT BITES

 Prevention

When you are in wooded or grassy areas:

- Wear a long-sleeved shirt and long pants.
- Tuck your pant legs into your socks or boots and tuck your shirt into your pants. In areas with ticks, use a rubber band or tape the area where your pants meet your socks so that nothing can get underneath.
- Wear light-coloured clothing to make it easier to see tiny insects or ticks.

- Don't wear perfume.
- When you are hiking in woods and fields, stay in the middle of trails.
- Stay away from underbrush and tall grass.
- Check yourself carefully for insects or ticks after you get inside.
- If you have pets that go outdoors, spray them with repellent made for your type of pet. Check them for ticks and insects often because your pet can bring these into your home.

▶ What to Look For

- Pain, redness, or swelling at the site of the injury
- Insects nearby

What to Do

Check:

- Check the scene to ensure it is safe.
- If it is safe to do so, check the person and the person's ABCs.

Call:

- Call EMS/9-1-1 and get an AED if there are any signs of a severe allergic reaction.

Care:

NOTE:

Not all insects leave a stinger embedded in the skin. For example, ants don't.

 1 Ensure the person's ABCs are present.

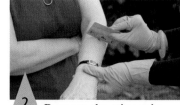

2 Remove the stinger by scraping it away from the skin.

3 Perform a secondary survey and treat any non-life-threatening conditions:

- Wash the area with soap and water.
- Apply a cold pack to help control swelling but put a thin cloth between the cold pack and the person's skin to avoid freezing the skin.

4 Watch for signs of an allergic reaction (see Chapter 6).

If you use an insect repellent, don't use it around your lips, eyes, or any wounds or irritated skin. Follow the instructions on the label carefully. When you come inside, wash your skin with soap and water to remove the repellent. With children, do not use any insect repellents with diethyltoluamide (DEET) in concentrations greater than 25 percent.

TICK BITES

 What to Do

Check:

- Check the scene to ensure it is safe.
- If it is safe to do so, check the person and the person's ABCs.

Call:

- There is no need to call EMS/9-1-1 and get an AED for a tick bite.

Care:

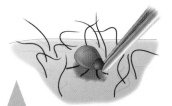

▲ **1** Ensure the person's ABCs are present.

▲ **2** If the tick hasn't started to dig into the flesh, remove it by brushing it off the skin.

▲ **3** If the tick has started to dig into the flesh, grasp its head with tweezers and pull it out.

▲ **4** Perform a secondary survey and treat any non-life-threatening conditions:

- When the tick is out, wash the area with soap and water. Then apply an antiseptic or antibiotic ointment to prevent infection, after checking the Five Rights of Medication.
- If you cannot remove the tick or if its mouthparts stay in the skin, seek medical attention.

▲ **5** If a rash or flu-like symptoms appear within a month after the tick bite, seek medical attention. See "**Lyme Disease**" on page 170.

LYME DISEASE

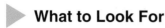 ### Causes

- A bite from an infected tick

 ### What to Look For

Early symptoms:

- A rash in a small red area that spreads up to 13–18 cm (5–7 in.) across
- Fever, headache, weakness, and joint and muscle pain that may feel like the flu

Later symptoms (weeks or months after the bite):

- Arthritis, numbness, or a stiff neck
- Memory loss
- Problems seeing or hearing
- A high fever
- An irregular or rapid heartbeat

 ### What to Do

Seek medical attention as soon as possible.

STINGS FROM MARINE LIFE

NOTE:

None of the sea urchins in Canada are poisonous. Poisonous sea urchins can be found in other parts of the world.

In Canada, stings from marine life are usually from jellyfish. In other parts of the world, animals such as stingrays and sea urchins can sting you when in the water.

 ### Prevention

Know the water you are swimming in and stay away from stinging marine life.

 ### What to Look For

- Pain
- Rash
- Redness
- Swelling

 ### What to Do

Check:

- Check the scene to ensure it is safe.
- If it is safe to do so, check the person and the person's ABCs.

Call:

- Call EMS/9-1-1 and get an AED if the person is having airway or breathing problems.

Care:

1. Ensure the person's ABCs are present.

2. Wash the area with vinegar for at least 30 seconds. If vinegar isn't available, use a mixture of baking soda and water (to make a consistency like toothpaste) and leave it on the area for 20 minutes. Then immerse the affected area in hot water (as tolerated) for 20 minutes or as long as the pain persists. Do not rub the area.

3. While wearing gloves, remove any tentacles or pieces of the animal.

4. Scrape or shave the area with a razor or the edge of a knife.

5. Perform a secondary survey and treat any non-life-threatening conditions:

   - Put a cold pack on the area for the first hour to reduce the pain.

6. After the area dries, apply a cream as recommended by a pharmacist after checking the Five Rights of Medication.

> **NOTE:**
> Remember your gloves and other barrier devices.

SNAKEBITES

 Prevention

- Do not aggravate a snake.
- If out hiking, watch where you are stepping.
- Wear proper footwear when hiking.

 What to Do

Check:

- Check the scene to ensure it is safe.
- If it is safe to do so, check the person and the person's ABCs.

Call:

- Call EMS/9-1-1 and get an AED.

Care:

1. Ensure the person's ABCs are present.

2. Keep the injured site still and lower than the heart if possible.

> **NOTE:**
> Remember your gloves and other barrier devices.

3. Perform a secondary survey and treat any non-life-threatening conditions:

- Check the temperature and colour of the limb beyond the site of the bite and note if it is abnormally cold or warm compared to the other limb. Report this to EMS personnel.

- If you have a physical description of the snake, report it to EMS personnel because it may help them provide the best treatment.

Never treat snakebites by:

- Applying ice
- Applying suction
- Cutting the wound
- Applying a tourniquet

ANIMAL BITES

 What to Do

Check:

- Check the scene to ensure it is safe.
- If it is safe to do so, check the person and the person's ABCs.

Call:

- Call your local animal control department.

Care:

1. Try to get the person safely away from the animal without injuring yourself.
2. Do not try to capture the animal.
3. Ensure the person's ABCs are present.
4. Control any deadly bleeding.
5. Perform a secondary survey and treat any non-life-threatening conditions.

NOTE:

If the animal is not familiar to you or there is severe bleeding, seek medical attention.

If the wound is minor:

- Wash it with soap and water.
- Control any bleeding and put a dressing on the wound.

6. Watch later for signs and symptoms of infection (see Chapter 8).

SUBSTANCE MISUSE AND ABUSE

Many substances, such as alcohol and drugs, can be used improperly (Figure 13.1). When these substances are misused or abused, they poison the body.

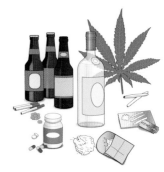

Figure 13.1 Alcohol and drugs.

Stimulants

- Stimulants affect your brain and nerves to speed up physical and mental activity.

- Many stimulants are taken as pills, but some can be absorbed or inhaled.

Hallucinogens

- Hallucinogens cause changes in mood, sensation, thought, emotion, and self-awareness.

- They can cause intense fear, panic, paranoid delusions, vivid hallucinations, deep depression, tension, and anxiety.

Depressants

- Depressants send signals to your brain and nerves that slow down physical and mental activity.

- They make you drowsy and impair your coordination and judgment.

- Alcohol is the most widely used and abused depressant in Canada.

Designer Drugs

- Designer drugs do not fit into any of the categories mentioned above.

- They are chemically altered versions of medical drugs, such as **narcotics** and amphetamines.

- The effects can be unpredictable and dangerous.

- One of the more commonly used designer drugs is "Ecstasy."

What to Look For

Like other poisons, the general signs and symptoms of substance misuse and abuse are similar to those of other medical emergencies:

- Moist or flushed skin
- Chills or fever
- Changes in breathing
- Changes in the level of consciousness
- Sweating
- Nausea or vomiting
- Seizures
- Altered mental status

What to Do

Check:

• Check the scene to ensure it is safe.

• If it is safe to do so, check the person and the person's ABCs.

Call:

• Call EMS/9-1-1 and get an AED if the person is having seizures, has difficulty breathing, is unconscious, or is behaving aggressively.

> **NOTE:**
>
> Remember your gloves and other barrier devices.

> **NOTE:**
>
> **For Healthcare Providers:** You can also check for an abnormal pulse.

Care:

1. Ensure the person's ABCs are present.

2. Perform a secondary survey and treat any non-life-threatening conditions:

   • You don't need to know exactly what substance the person has taken. Just look for any abnormal:

   ▶ Breathing

   ▶ Skin colour, temperature, and moisture

   ▶ Behaviour

3. Provide continual care.

ALCOHOL POISONING

Alcohol impairs your judgment, slows down your reflexes, and makes driving unsafe. Just two drinks in less than an hour can create unsafe levels of alcohol in the blood of an average 72.5 kilogram (160-pound) person.

Alcohol poisoning is a condition in which a toxic amount of alcohol has entered the body.

 Causes

• Drinking excessive amounts of alcohol in a short period of time

> **Prevention**
>
> • Have non-alcoholic beverages available at a party.
>
> • Limit yourself to one drink per hour.
>
> • Don't drink before a party.
>
> • If you are angry or depressed, refrain from drinking alcohol.

- Eat plenty of food before you drink and while you are drinking.
- Avoid salty foods that may make you thirsty and encourage you to drink more.
- Do not play drinking games.

▶ What to Look For

- Confusion
- Seizures
- Low body temperature
- Blue-tinged skin or skin that is paler than normal

- Vomiting
- Slow or irregular breathing
- Unconsciousness

What to Do

Check:

- Check the scene to ensure it is safe.
- If it is safe to do so, check the person and the person's ABCs.

Call:

- Have someone call EMS/9-1-1 and get an AED. If you are alone, call EMS/9-1-1 yourself, get an AED, and then return to care for the person.

Care:

1. Ensure the person's ABCs are present.
2. Perform a secondary survey and treat any non-life-threatening conditions.
3. Roll the person into the recovery position.

NOTES:

Additional Skills for Healthcare Providers

Additional Skills for Healthcare Providers

You and your partner receive a call to assist at a community swimming pool, where a boy has been pulled from the water after hitting his head on the diving board. He's unconscious and not breathing. When you arrive, you find a lifeguard administering CPR. She says she's been doing so for about eight minutes, with no sign of response.

Healthcare providers are generally those who have a duty to respond to an emergency medical incident as a team and often include physicians, nurses, allied healthcare professionals, and first responders such as paramedics and firefighters. These personnel are often the first trained professionals to arrive at the scene of an emergency and are required to learn additional CPR/AED skills outlined in this chapter.

JAW THRUST

If you think a person might have a head and/or spine injury, use a **jaw thrust** to open the airway instead of a head-tilt/chin-lift:

> **NOTE:**
>
> If you cannot keep the airway open with a jaw thrust, use the head-tilt/chin-lift. Remember, it is important to keep an open airway and get air in.

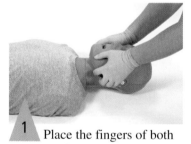

1 Place the fingers of both hands on the angles of the jaw.

2 Lift the jaw forward while keeping gentle pressure on the cheeks to keep the head from moving off the ground.

3 Place the mask over the person's mouth and nose.

4 Give two breaths/ventilations. Each breath should last one second, with just enough volume to make the chest start to rise.

HOW TO DO A PULSE CHECK

▶ Adult or Child

During your ABC check, you can do a pulse check to assess circulation. To check the carotid pulse of an adult or child:

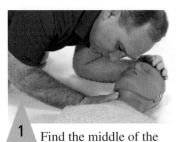

2 Slide your fingers into the groove at the side of the neck closest to you.

1 Find the middle of the person's throat (Adam's apple).

▶ Baby

To check the brachial pulse of a baby:

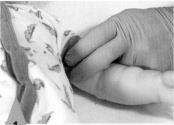

2 Gently push in against the upper arm bone. Keep your thumb off the arm.

1 Place one or two fingers on the underside of the baby's arm halfway between the elbow and the shoulder.

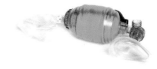

> **NOTE:**
>
> The pulse may be hard to find if it is slow or weak. If after a maximum of 5 to 10 seconds you are not certain there is a pulse, start CPR.

> **NOTE:**
>
> If the pulse of an unresponsive child or baby is less than 60 beats per minute (bpm) and there are signs of poor perfusion (pallor cyanosis), begin chest compressions.

Figure 14.1 A bag-valve-mask.

BAG-VALVE-MASK

- A **bag-valve-mask (BVM)** has three parts: a bag, a valve, and a mask. They need to be put together before you can use the BVM (Figure 14.1).

- You must have two rescuers to use a BVM:

  ▶ One rescuer opens the person's airway with a head-tilt/chin-lift and/or jaw thrust and puts the mask on the person's face, making sure there is a tight seal.

  ▶ The second rescuer squeezes the bag (Figure 14.2). Much like rescue breathing, the bag should be squeezed smoothly, not forcefully, with just enough volume to make the chest start to rise.

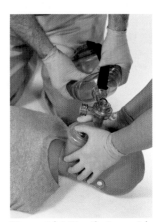

Figure 14.2 Ventilations with a BVM.

RESCUE BREATHING

 What to Do

Two-Rescuer Rescue Breathing for an Adult or Child

Check:

- Check the scene to ensure it is safe.

- If it is safe to do so, check the person and the person's ABCs.

Call:

- If the person does not respond, have someone call EMS/9-1-1 and get an AED.

Care:

> **NOTE:**
>
> If the person is face down and breathing cannot be assessed, roll the person over to assess breathing.

1. If you do not hear normal breathing, give two rescue breaths/ventilations:

   - One rescuer opens the person's airway with a head-tilt/chin-lift and/or jaw thrust and puts the mask on the person's face, making sure there is a tight seal.

   - The second rescuer squeezes the bag. Much like rescue breathing, the bag should be squeezed smoothly, not forcefully, with just enough volume to make the chest start to rise.

2. If there is a pulse, continue rescue breathing:

   - For an adult, give one breath/ventilation every five to six seconds.

   - For a child, give one breath/ventilation every three to five seconds.

3. After two minutes of rescue breathing, check again for signs of circulation and normal breathing for no longer than 5 to 10 seconds:

   - Look for chest rise, movement, coughing, breathing, and abnormal skin colour (e.g., pale, bluish appearance, etc.).

   - Feel for a carotid pulse.

4. If there are signs of circulation and breathing, perform a secondary survey and treat any non-life-threatening conditions.

5. If there are signs of circulation but no breathing, continue rescue breathing.

6. If there are no signs of circulation, perform CPR.

7. Provide continual care until EMS personnel arrive.

Two-Rescuer Rescue Breathing for a Baby

Check:

- Check the scene to ensure it is safe.
- If it is safe to do so, check the baby and the baby's ABCs.

Call:

- If the baby does not respond, have someone call EMS/9-1-1 and get an AED.

Care:

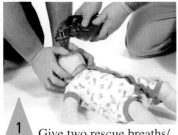

1 Give two rescue breaths/ventilations:

- One rescuer places the mask over the baby's mouth and nose, making sure there is a tight seal.
- The second rescuer gives two breaths/ventilations, each lasting one second, with just enough volume to make the chest start to rise.

2 If there is a pulse, continue rescue breathing:

- Give the baby one breath/ventilation every three to five seconds.

3 After two minutes of rescue breathing, check again for signs of circulation and normal breathing for no more than 5 to 10 seconds:

- Look for chest rise, movement, coughing, breathing, and abnormal skin colour.
- Feel for a brachial pulse.

4 If there are signs of circulation and breathing, perform a secondary survey and treat any non-life-threatening conditions.

5 If there are signs of circulation but no breathing, continue rescue breathing.

NOTE:

When performing the head-tilt/chin-lift on a baby, do not tilt the head back too far.

6 If there are no signs of circulation, perform CPR.

7 Provide continual care until EMS personnel arrive.

TWO-RESCUER CPR

 ## Two-Rescuer CPR for an Adult or Child

Two rescuers can work together to give CPR to an adult or child:

1. One rescuer begins CPR while the second rescuer calls EMS/9-1-1 and gets an AED.

2. When the second rescuer returns, one rescuer performs chest compressions and gives rescue breaths/ventilations. The other rescuer maintains the head-tilt/chin-lift and/or jaw thrust with the BVM.

3. For an adult, use the same technique and ratios as in adult CPR with one rescuer (30 compressions to 2 breaths/ventilations). For a child, when there are two rescuers, use a ratio of 15 compressions to 2 breaths/ventilations.

4. Switch with the other rescuer every two minutes (between cycles) to maintain the quality of CPR.

5. Continue CPR until the AED arrives.

For the purpose of all first aid, *except* when using an AED, a child is considered as being between one year old and the onset of puberty.

Two-Rescuer CPR for a Baby

Two rescuers can also work together to give CPR to a baby:

1. One rescuer begins CPR while the second rescuer calls EMS/9-1-1 and gets an AED.

2. When the second rescuer returns, one rescuer performs chest compressions and gives rescue breaths/ventilations while the other rescuer maintains the head-tilt/chin-lift and/or jaw thrust with the BVM. Use a ratio of 15 compressions to 2 breaths/ventilations.

3. Switch with the other rescuer every two minutes (between cycles) to maintain the quality of CPR.

4. Continue CPR until the AED arrives.

Alternate method: One rescuer maintains the head-tilt/ chin-lift and/or jaw thrust, while the second rescuer encircles the baby's chest with both hands, spreading his or her fingers around the baby's back and placing both thumbs on the lower half of the baby's breastbone. While the first rescuer maintains the head-tilt/chin-lift and/or jaw thrust, the second rescuer gives rescue breaths/ventilations, maintaining a ratio of 15 compressions to 2 breaths/ventilations.

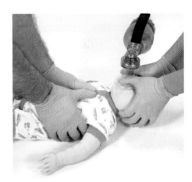

NOTES:

Kit Contents

Kit Contents

EXAMPLE OF A FIRST AID KIT

Keep a first aid kit readily available in your home, cottage, car, boat, workplace, and recreation area (Figure A.1). Store it in a dry place and replace used or outdated contents regularly.

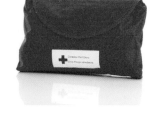

Figure A.1 A first aid kit.

A first aid kit should contain the following:

❏ Emergency telephone numbers for EMS, your local Poison Control Centre, and your personal doctors

❏ Home and office phone numbers for family members, friends, or neighbours who can help

❏ Sterile gauze pads (dressings) in small and large squares to place over wounds

❏ Adhesive tape

❏ Roller and triangular bandages to hold dressings in place or to make an arm sling

❏ Adhesive bandages in assorted sizes

❏ Scissors

❏ Tweezers

❏ Safety pins

❏ Instant ice packs

❏ Disposable non-latex gloves, such as surgical or examination gloves

❏ Flashlight, with extra batteries in a separate bag

❏ Antiseptic wipes, soap, and hand sanitizer

❏ Pencil and pad

❏ Emergency blanket

❏ Eye patches

❏ Thermometer

❏ Barrier devices, such as a pocket mask or face shield

❏ Coins for pay phone

❏ Canadian Red Cross *First Aid & CPR Manual*

For more information on the different types of Canadian Red Cross first aid kits that are available, please contact your local Red Cross office or look on our website at www.redcross.ca.

NOTE:

Legislation dictates what type of first aid kit is required for the workplace. Go to www.redcross.ca/firstaidlegislation for more details.

EXAMPLE OF AN EMERGENCY SUPPLIES KIT

Have supplies ready for an emergency. Store them in a backpack or a duffle bag so you can take them with you if you have to evacuate the area.

- ❏ Four litres (one gallon) of water per person per day (use sealed, unbreakable containers and replace the supply every six months). Have enough for at least three days.
- ❏ Packaged or canned food that won't go bad and a can opener. Replace the food once a year.
- ❏ Walking shoes, rain gear, and a change of clothing
- ❏ Blankets or sleeping bags
- ❏ A first aid kit and prescription medications (check the medications every six months to make sure they haven't passed their expiry date)
- ❏ Toilet paper and other personal supplies
- ❏ An extra pair of glasses
- ❏ A battery-powered radio and flashlight, along with extra batteries
- ❏ Spare cash
- ❏ An extra set of car keys
- ❏ A list of your family doctors
- ❏ Important family information such as a list of any medical conditions or medical devices, such as pacemakers
- ❏ Photocopies of all important identification for you and your family, including health card numbers
- ❏ Special items for babies, elderly, or disabled household members
- ❏ Cellphone and contact information for family and friends

EXAMPLE OF AN EMERGENCY CAR KIT

Keep an emergency kit in your car.

❏ A battery-powered radio and flashlight, with extra batteries

❏ A blanket

❏ Booster (jumper) cables

❏ A fire extinguisher

❏ A Canadian Red Cross first aid kit

❏ Bottled water and non-perishable high-energy foods (replace the water every six months and the food once a year)

❏ Maps of the area

❏ A shovel

❏ Flares

❏ A tire repair kit and pump

❏ Matches and a "survival" candle in a deep can that will burn for many hours

Glossary

ABCs: Airway, breathing, and circulation.

Abdomen: The part of the body below the chest and above the pelvis. It contains the stomach, intestines, liver, spleen, and other organs.

Abdominal thrusts: A method to remove a foreign object from the airway.

Absorbed poison: A poison that enters the body through the skin.

Airway: The pathway for air from the mouth and nose to the lungs.

Airway obstruction: Something in the airway that stops air from reaching the lungs.

Allergic reaction: The body's response to a substance to which it is particularly sensitive. The response can be mild or very severe.

Amputation: The complete or partial severing of a body part.

Anaphylaxis: A severe allergic reaction.

Anemia: A condition caused by a lack of red blood cells.

Angina: A cardiovascular condition in which the heart muscles need more oxygen than they are getting, causing chest pain or pressure that comes and goes. It is usually more frequent with exertion or stress.

Arteries: Large blood vessels that carry oxygen-rich blood from the heart to the rest of the body.

Aspiration: Inhaling blood, vomit, saliva, or foreign material into the lungs.

Asthma: A condition that narrows the air passages and makes breathing difficult. Asthma is more common in children.

Automated External Defibrillator (AED): An electronic device that analyzes the heart's electrical rhythm and, if necessary, tells the user to deliver a shock to a person in cardiac arrest.

Baby: A child up to one year of age.

Bag-valve-mask (BVM): A hand-held device used to ventilate a non-breathing person. It has three parts: a bag, a valve, and a mask.

Bandage: Material used to wrap or cover a part of the body or to hold a dressing or splint in place.

Bone: The dense, hard tissue that forms the skeleton.

Brain: The centre of the nervous system that controls body functions.

Breathing emergency: A situation in which breathing is so impaired that the person's life is in danger.

Burn: An injury caused by heat, chemicals, electricity, or radiation.

Bystander: Someone who is present at the scene of a situation or emergency.

Cardiac arrest: A condition in which the heart has stopped beating or beats too irregularly or too weakly to pump blood effectively.

Cardiopulmonary resuscitation (CPR): A first aid technique that combines rescue breaths and chest compressions for someone whose breathing and heart have stopped.

Cardiovascular disease: Any disease of the heart and blood vessels. Also called heart disease.

Care: A check and immediate treatment for conditions that are an immediate threat to someone's life.

Cells: The basic units of all living tissue.

Check, Call, Care: The basic steps to follow in any emergency.

Chest thrusts: An alternate method to remove a foreign object from the airway.

Child: Anyone between the ages of one and eight. (One to the onset of puberty for healthcare providers except when using an AED.)

Choking: The condition in which someone's airway is partly or completely blocked by a foreign object.

Cholesterol: A fatty substance that can cause buildup on artery walls, making the arteries narrower and restricting blood flow.

Cold-related emergency: A general term for conditions caused by being exposed to cold temperatures for too long. Includes frost nip, frostbite, and hypothermia.

Compression: Rhythmic pressure that is put on the chest to dislodge something blocking the airway or to circulate blood when the heart isn't beating effectively.

Concussion: A temporary impairment of brain function, usually caused by a blow to the head.

Conscious: A state of awareness and responsiveness.

Consent: The permission given by the ill or injured person to the First Aider to provide care.

Continual care: Providing reassurance and follow-up care after an injury or illness.

Contraction: A squeezing action made by the muscles in the womb during labour, in preparation for childbirth.

Crush injury: An injury caused when a crushing force is applied to any part of the body over a short or long period of time.

Defibrillation: An electric shock that is given to correct a life-threatening heart rhythm.

Diabetes: A condition in which a person cannot regulate the balance between insulin and sugar.

Diabetic emergency: A condition in which a person with diabetes becomes ill because of a blood sugar level that is too high or too low.

Direct pressure: Pressure that is put on a wound to control bleeding.

Disease: An impairment of health or a condition of abnormal functioning.

Disease transmission (direct contact, indirect contact, airborne, vector-borne): The four different ways that infections can be spread from one person to another.

Dislocation: An injury in which a bone is moved out of its normal position at a joint.

Dispatcher: The emergency medical services person who answers the emergency telephone number and decides which EMS professionals to send to the scene and who may give advice about first aid until EMS personnel arrive.

Dressing: A pad placed directly over a wound to absorb blood and other body fluids and to prevent infection.

Elevate: A technique to help slow the flow of blood to an injured area, such as a fracture, by raising the injured body part above the level of the heart.

Emergency: A situation requiring immediate action.

Emergency medical services (EMS) personnel: Trained and equipped people, including police, firefighters, and ambulance personnel, who are dispatched through a local emergency number to give emergency care to ill or injured people.

Emergency medical services (EMS) system: A network of community resources and personnel organized to give emergency care in cases of injury or sudden illness.

Epinephrine: A drug that can be injected into the body to counteract a severe allergic reaction.

Erectile dysfunction drugs: Prescription medications such as Viagra®, Levitra®, and Cialis®, used to treat problems getting or maintaining an erection.

Exhaling: To breathe air out of the lungs.

External bleeding: Bleeding from an open wound in the skin.

Fainting: A loss of consciousness caused by a temporary drop in blood flow to the brain.

First aid: Immediate care given to someone who is ill or injured until more advanced care can be obtained.

First Aider: A person with some training who gives immediate care to someone who is ill or injured until more advanced care can be obtained.

Flail chest: An injury involving multiple fractured ribs that, as a result, do not move normally with the rest of the chest during breathing.

Foreign object: Any item that enters a body from outside; most common foreign objects enter a person's eyes, ears, nose, airway, or rectum.

Fracture: A break in bone tissue.

Frostbite: The freezing of the skin and underlying tissues of a particular body part. It is a serious condition that most often affects the fingers, toes, ears, and nose.

Frost nip: The freezing of the skin of a particular body part. It is a superficial injury that most often affects the fingers, toes, ears, and nose.

Full-thickness burn: A burn that affects both layers of skin and the tissues underneath. The skin may be charred. Also known as a third-degree burn.

H.A.IN.E.S. recovery position: A recovery position for an unconscious person. This position helps to keep the airway open and allows any blood or vomit to drain from the person's mouth.

Hands-off check: A survey of a conscious, responsive person's injuries that combines visual observation and questions and answers.

Hands-on check: A check of injuries for an unconscious person or a person with an altered level of consciousness. It involves physically examining the person and monitoring the person's vital signs.

Head-tilt/chin-lift: A technique for opening the airway in an unconscious adult, child, or baby.

Head-to-toe check: A thorough check for injuries or conditions that need attention and could become life-threatening or limb-threatening if they are not cared for.

Heart: The muscular organ that pumps blood through the body.

Heart attack: A sudden illness in which an artery that feeds the heart becomes blocked, stopping part of the heart muscle from getting the oxygen-rich blood that it needs.

Heat cramps: Muscle pains, usually involving the calf and abdominal muscles, caused by working or exercising in a hot environment.

Heat exhaustion: A condition that occurs when the body temperature gets too high, usually from hard work or exercise in a hot, humid environment.

Heat-related emergency: A range of conditions caused when the body temperature gets too high, usually from hard work or exercise in a hot, humid environment. It includes heat cramps, heat exhaustion, and heat stroke.

Heat stroke: A life-threatening condition that develops when the body's temperature is extremely high and the body cannot cool itself.

Hemothorax: A condition in which blood accumulates in the chest cavity from the wound site but doesn't get into the lung. Because blood takes up space in the chest cavity, the lung can't expand effectively.

Heredity: The passing of physical or mental traits from one generation to the next through genetics.

Hyperglycemia: A diabetic condition in which there is too much sugar in the bloodstream.

Hyperventilation: A condition that occurs when breathing is faster than normal, upsetting the body's balance of oxygen and carbon dioxide.

Hypoglycemia: A diabetic condition in which there is too little sugar in the bloodstream.

Hypothermia: A life-threatening condition that develops when the body's temperature drops too low, usually from being exposed to cold temperatures for too long.

Immobilize: To use a splint or other method to keep an injured body part from moving.

Immunization: The introduction of a substance into the body that builds up a person's resistance against the germs that cause a specific disease.

Impaled object: An object remaining in a wound.

Infection: A condition caused by germs such as viruses and bacteria.

Inhale: To breathe into the lungs.

Inhaled poison: A poison that is breathed into the lungs.

Inhaler: A portable device used for administering a medicinal gas or vapour.

Injected poison: A poison that enters the body through a bite, sting, or hypodermic needle.

Injury: Damage to the body from an external force such as a blow, fall, fire, or collision.

Insulin: A hormone the body needs to use sugar for energy.

Internal bleeding: Bleeding inside the body.

Jaw thrust: An alternative to the head-tilt/chin-lift method for opening the airway.

Joint: Where two or more bones meet.

Labour: The contractions of the womb that come before childbirth.

Ligament: A fibrous band that holds bones together at a joint.

Lungs: The pair of organs that take oxygen in and remove carbon dioxide during breathing.

Lyme disease: An illness spread by infected ticks.

MedicAlert® medical identification product: A wallet card or a bracelet, watch strap, anklet, or necklace with a tag indicating that the person wearing it has a particular medical condition.

Medical emergency: An illness or condition requiring immediate medical attention.

Muscle: A soft tissue that lengthens and shortens to move body parts.

Narcotics: A group of drugs that reduces pain and induces sleep.

Nerve: A part of the nervous system that carries impulses between the brain and all body parts.

Nitroglycerin: A medication often prescribed to people diagnosed with angina.

Normal breathing: A state when airways to the lungs are fully open, allowing air to easily move in and out.

Osteoporosis: A bone disease characterized by reduced bone mass and density, which results in brittle bones that easily fracture. It is a leading cause of bone and joint injuries in older people.

Partial-thickness burn: A burn through both layers of skin. The skin may blister and look red and wet. Sometimes called a second-degree burn.

Pelvis: The part of the body between the abdomen and the legs. It contains the intestines, bladder, and reproductive organs.

Pneumothorax: A condition in which air enters the chest cavity from the wound site, but doesn't enter the lung. The air in the chest cavity presses against the lung, causing it to collapse.

Poison: Any substance that causes injury, illness, or death when it enters the body.

Poison Control Centre: A centre staffed by medical professionals to give information about first aid in cases of poisoning. Poison Control Centre phone numbers are on the inside front page of the telephone directory.

Primary survey: An examination of the emergency scene and the ill or injured person for life-threatening conditions.

Pulse: The beat felt in arteries near the skin with each contraction of the heart.

Radiation burn: A burn caused by rays, energy, or electromagnetic waves.

Rescue breathing: The technique of breathing air into someone who isn't breathing.

Respiratory arrest: A condition in which breathing has stopped or isn't effective.

Respiratory distress: A condition in which breathing is difficult.

Risk factors: Conditions or behaviours that increase the chance that a person will develop a particular disease or get a particular injury.

Secondary survey: A verbal, visual, and physical check of an ill or injured person for conditions that need attention and could become life-threatening if they are not cared for.

Seizures: Episodes of abnormal electrical signals in the brain that result in disturbed brain function, shaking or contraction of limbs, and altered consciousness.

Self-administration of medication: A person giving himself or herself a dose of medication orally or through an injector or inhaler.

Shaken Baby Syndrome (SBS): The type of injuries or combination of injuries a baby or child receives from being shaken.

Shock: A serious condition caused when the circulatory system cannot get enough oxygen-rich blood to all parts of the body. It can be the result of severe blood loss or an allergic reaction, among other causes.

Sign: A signal of injury or illness that a First Aider can see, feel, smell, or hear.

Skin: The membrane that covers the entire surface of the body.

Soft tissue: The layers of skin, fat, muscles, and other soft body structures.

Splint: A device used to stop body parts from moving.

Sprain: The stretching and tearing of ligaments and other soft tissues at a joint.

Stoma: An opening in the front of the neck through which a person can breathe.

Strain: The stretching and tearing of muscles and tendons.

Stroke: A disruption of blood flow in the brain, causing weakness and/or speech problems.

Superficial burn: A burn that affects just the top layer of skin. The skin will look red and dry. Sometimes called a first-degree burn.

Swallowed (ingested) poison: A poison that enters the body by being swallowed.

Symptom: A signal of injury or illness that the ill or injured person tells you that he or she feels.

Tendon: A fibrous band that attaches muscle to bone.

Tissue: A group of cells that work together to perform specific functions.

Transient ischemic attack (TIA): A temporary drop in blood flow to part of the brain; sometimes called a mini-stroke.

Triage: The process of sorting and providing care to several ill or injured people according to the severity of their injuries or illnesses.

Unconscious: Describing the state of a person who is unaware of the surrounding environment and is unresponsive to stimuli.

Veins: Blood vessels that carry oxygen-poor blood from all parts of the body back to the heart.

Vertebrae: The 33 bones that make up the spine.

Vital signs: Three key characteristics of someone's condition: level of consciousness, breathing, and the appearance of the skin.

Wound: An injury to soft tissues.

Index